The Girl on the Shore

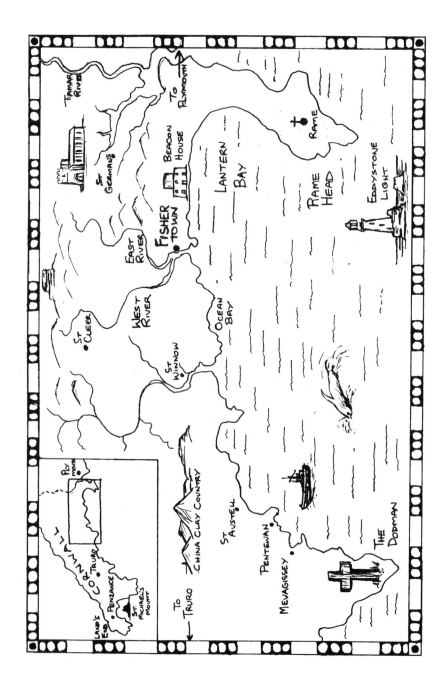

The Girl on the Shore

Adventures at Beacon House – A Care Home with a Difference

F. M. Hughes

Jessica Kingsley Publishers
London and Philadelphia

First published in the United Kingdom in 2003
by Jessica Kingsley Publishers Ltd
116 Pentonville Road
London N1 9JB, England
and
325 Chestnut Street
Philadelphia, PA 19106, USA

www.jkp.com

Library of Congress Cataloging in Publication Data
A CIP catalog record for this book is available from the Library of Congress

British Library Cataloguing in Publication Data
A CIP catalogue record for this book is available from the British Library

ISBN 1 84310 111 4

Printed and Bound in Great Britain by
Athenaeum Press, Gateshead, Tyne and Wear

Contents

To Kay and Inky

F. M. Hughes is a psychologist with many years' experience of working with older people. The Hughes family go sailing together every summer.

The queue of people wanting late breakfast and mid-morning snacks just hadn't stopped. It must be the warmer weather of early spring that was bringing them out. And now there was this old man at the front of the queue who couldn't make up his mind. He dithered at the long list of choices on the menu. "What do you think I should have?" he asked. Gemma could see the people behind him getting restless but she ignored them and only paid attention to him. She suggested tea and a scone, or would he prefer coffee? "No, definitely tea and that scone" he said, relieved at having made the decision. As he went off to one of the empty seats, Gemma thought she noticed a smartly dressed, middle-aged woman watching her.

After he'd drunk his tea, the old man asked for the bill. She brought it to him and, after much rummaging in his bag, he produced a purse and offered it to her. She carefully opened it and placed the coins on the table, counting them aloud till they reached the required amount. And as she did so, she was again aware that the woman was watching her. At last things calmed down a bit and she went round the tables to give them a wipe. A newspaper lay open at the table where the woman had been sitting. It was the Jobs Vacant page and one advertisement had been neatly circled in red ink. She briefly glanced at it: "Beacon House, Lantern Beach: extra support worker wanted. Full-time. Training provided for the right person. A permanent and rewarding post." Picking up the newspaper, she put it in the binbag she was carrying around with her as she tidied up.

Chapter One

Beginnings

On Lantern Beach

On the brow of the hill, she got off her bike, and took in the view. To the east, the land arced round to rise to the triangular headland of Rame, with its chapel silhouetted black by the sun; to the west, she saw the pier and the seafront of Fishertown where she had cycled from this morning; and, further away, a long arm of land ran far out into the sea: the great headland of the Dodman. Beneath her, the cliffs dropped away till they were replaced by dunes of light sand that were ever moving and flickering in the wind. Then came a grassy strip before the beach stretched down to the sea. The restless blue-green sea was flecked by the white tops of wind-driven waves that rolled onto Lantern Beach.

She stood for a while, enjoying the great sweep of seascape, until her reverie was broken by the honking and wing flaps of a small V-shaped flock of wild geese coming in from the sea; and a voice inside her head said sternly: "You mustn't be late for your interview".

She got back on her bike, and cycled down the steep road between the sandhills. She had to use her feet to brake on the bends, down and on down, till the road flattened and ran along the strip of green at the top of the beach.

Coming round the last bend, she saw a large, whitewashed building standing alone at the eastern end of the beach. It must be Beacon House.

She placed her bike against the outside of the garden wall, walked across the grass to the front door and rang the bell.

The door was opened by a middle-aged lady in a summery dress. "Welcome. I'm Rose and you must be Gemma who's come about the job. Matron – Muriel – Mrs O'Halloran – is expecting you." She led Gemma into the building. She knocked on a door but did not wait for an answer before opening it and beckoning Gemma to go in.

An older, thin woman with grey hair was working at a desk. Gemma realized at first with surprise, but then was not really surprised, that Mrs O'Halloran was the same woman who had been watching her in the café that time. She now put down her pen and turned to look over her glasses at Gemma. She rose and shook Gemma's hand. "Thank you for coming all this way. Do sit down. I expect you'd like a cup of tea?"

Gemma wanted to say "Thank you" but somehow the words just wouldn't come out of her mouth. She blushed, and gave a nod, instead of words. She imagined how the Matron – whom she so wanted to impress – must surely be seeing her, as a slightly large, big-boned, short-haired, round-faced teenager.

When she had put the kettle on, Mrs O'Halloran said, "Well, welcome to Beacon House, although everyone round here just calls it the Beacon. The beach ends at Beacon Point, which might have been used as a signal fire for events – like sighting the Armada–", she smiled "–but more likely was used by smugglers to guide in their boats with contraband brandy."

She poured out two cups from a china teapot with a rose petal design and gave Gemma a matching cup and saucer. Mrs O'Halloran sat down in a chair opposite her. "Well – would you like to tell me a bit about yourself?" she asked.

Gemma looked at her. What did the Matron want to know? What should she say that would make a good impression? And what would make a poor impression and lose her the chance of getting this job? That she was seventeen, and she had always lived in Fishertown – that was all right. But what should she say about her Dad? How much should she say about how her father had worked on the local boats, but hadn't been doing very well, so he'd gone down to Newlyn to work at the beam trawlers going deep-sea fishing; how his trips home had gradually become fewer and then stopped.

Her mother told her that he'd found someone else down there. Gemma had missed him at first and wondered if she'd done something to drive him away; but then he, and her feelings towards him, became a sort of emptiness. She had never done very well at school and left at sixteen without passing any proper exams. After she had left school, she'd worked the summer in a café near the pier; and after that, she'd only managed to find occasional work, till she had seen the advertisement for this job. But what parts of all this jumble, of bits of her life, should she talk about?

Mrs O'Halloran was looking at her. She had to say something, anything. So Gemma took the plunge and didn't try to leave bits out or make things sound better than they had been or than they were. And because Mrs O'Halloran seemed genuinely interested, she found it wasn't quite so hard telling her about her life.

"Thank you," said Mrs O'Halloran when Gemma had finished. "It's never easy talking about yourself, is it? Now I expect you want to hear something about the job you've come about.

"We're a residential unit for ten people. We're part of a national organization that was begun long ago as a religious foundation. We take in people who live locally. We want people to be able to stay here till they die. We want the residents to know that this is their home, however ill or infirm they may become on the way. That's why you'll find some of the staff are trained nurses, as I am myself. And what we also want to get across is that how much they enjoy living in their home will depend on how much each one of them puts into making it a good place to live – not just when they come in, but every day they're here."

She paused. "You're probably wondering how you might fit in; what–" she looked down at the copy of the advertisement on her desk "–an extra support worker actually does. Well, we want the residents to run this place as much as possible and to look after themselves and each other. So the menus are discussed and planned at our daily house meetings; and all the cooking is done by the residents, with the staff only providing help when needed; and when it's ready, everyone eats together and then helps with the washing up. During the day, we encourage them to do things they enjoy and feel good doing, perhaps picking up again on hobbies they haven't done for a while; and also to do things together, with and for each other. Some of the residents do this anyway, and we're just back-up. But obviously others come here because they do need more help, more encouragement and perhaps special resources or programmes. We have specialist staff who come here for sessions, but most of our staff are local people who haven't got any formal qualifications. What's important is that they're people who want to work in our way, and who show respect and warmth to our residents.

"So where would you fit into all this? Well, I think day-to-day, and across the days, we do well by our residents and they do well by us; but there are many times when a resident needs that bit of extra help; or wants to try something a bit different; or a couple of them want to go out, but all the staff are tied up, and so the opportunity – *that opportunity* for support or growth or adventure – is lost; and maybe next time the residents are less willing to try something new or different, so slowly they sink down; slowly they lose spirit…" Her voice tailed off as if – Gemma wondered – she was remembering some of those lost opportunities.

She gathered herself. "We *mustn't* lose those moments – which is where you come in. The purpose of your job will be to use the kindness I noticed in you that day in the café, to help the residents feel alive and growing. So, you will be available when staff spot the need for that bit of additional help that a resident can use."

She paused. "But all this probably doesn't mean very much to you yet. We'll talk some more as I show you around, but first, let's meet the residents." She looked at the clock on the wall. "Ten thirty – excellent. Coffee time."

They walked out of the office and into the living area of the home. It was an open space, off which were the bedrooms. "This first one is the room for staff who sleep in." Mrs O'Halloran pointed to the door of the next room. "When I told you we take ten people, that's the largest number we can take. In fact, early on, we decided to keep one bedroom for visitors, so that relatives could stay overnight if the resident wants them to; and at the moment, we have eight residents."

Three of the residents were making the coffee for everyone. "I've brought Gemma, who may be working with us soon. Can she join you?" Mrs O'Halloran asked.

"Sit you down," one of the ladies, who seemed rather thin, invited her. "I'm Mrs Bennett." She turned to an upright looking man opposite. "Corporal, would you be so good as to pop out and see if Tom or Beatrice want to join us?"

The coffee was brought over to a table in the lounge area which looked out south across the sea. Two members of staff – Rose and Barbara – sat down too. Barbara seemed about the same age as Rose. She wore a plain red dress, and seemed to worry if everyone and everything was all right a bit more than Rose did. The Corporal came back saying that Tom and Beatrice, as usual, wouldn't be coming up from the beach.

For a minute or two, Gemma felt alarmed. The faces of a few of the residents seemed to have shrunk so that they looked like the faces of skeletons barely covered by skin. Their skin was dry and lined. And she found it hard to think what to say to people who were so old and, she assumed, frail. She didn't like to ask the residents about themselves, in case they – or Mrs O'Halloran – thought she was being nosy. It should be all right to ask them where they had lived before coming to the Beacon, and they were happy to tell her. Mrs Bennett came from St Winnow on the Fowey River;

Mr Mitchell came from St Germans. He could only use one of his hands; the other hung down limp and lifeless. Gemma was to learn later he had had a stroke. The Corporal came from Talland. Mrs Austin was a tall, thin woman who seemed to have difficulty finding her words. With a bit of help from Barbara, it emerged she came from St Cleer "just down from the stone circles". George Meredith, a tall, thin man who seemed to pant and be short of breath, came from Lansallos.

After a quarter of an hour, Mrs O'Halloran rose. "We'll let you get on with the daily meeting. You remember the meeting on Friday gave me permission to miss today's, so that I can show Gemma around." Gemma thanked everyone for letting her have coffee with them.

As they walked off, Mrs O'Halloran explained about the daily meeting. It was where residents and staff could bring up anything of concern or interest. "It's an important part of the Beacon. And it works because we try to take people whilst they've still got the spirit – the desire to get something out of living, to take part and enjoy living here. If you wait too long, they may well have given up and started to turn their face to the wall, and away from people. Now let me show you our pride and joy – the Lookout."

They started going up the stairs. "There's a lift too, of course." At the top of the stairs, they entered a large circular room where the walls were all made of glass. Through them, Gemma could see the beaches and cliffs to the east and west and the sea stretching to the horizon.

"What a fantastic view!" she exclaimed.

"Yes," agreed Mrs O'Halloran, "It really is like being on the bridge of an ocean liner, isn't it? We've got a little bar, which is open at times residents want – like before lunch on weekends, and most days, early evenings. People like to sit here and watch the sun go down – the sunsets are just stunning. And they want their visitors or friends to see it too, so they bring them up for a drink; or they may just bring them up here at any time for a chat away from the others. You'll find they like to come up here to be by themselves." Gemma thought she too could spend hours up here just looking out at the sea.

"Well, Gemma." Mrs O'Halloran's voice cut into her thoughts. "What do you make of what you've seen so far?" Gemma took her eyes away from the view. She had lots of half-formed thoughts and feelings. She'd never worked or spent any time in a place like this. Her mother had taken her a few times to see Nan in a home before she died. They had walked down long corridors to a small room that smelt musty and had faded pictures on the wall; and Nan hadn't seemed to have kept hold of that spirit that Matron had been talking about. For months before she died, she used to take Gemma's hand and say "I hope my time comes soon" and Gemma hadn't known what to say.

It was time to answer *that* question. Her faltering reply was, "I would love to work here."

She had surprised herself. She didn't often let herself want things, because she usually didn't get them. "I'm glad," said Mrs O'Halloran. "I've got one or two more applicants to see, but I promise I'll let you know within the week."

As Gemma left, she saw that there were two people – a man and a woman – on different parts of the beach. Gemma supposed they must be Tom and Beatrice.

She picked up her bike and started homewards. Her movement brought up a small flock of oystercatchers that had been feeding on the low tide mark. They rose with a startled cry and flew rapidly away out to sea, their black and white plumage and long orange beaks picked out sharply above the blue sea.

She cycled back over the hills to Fishertown and then into the old part of town till she reached the small fisherman's cottage where she and her mother lived. She let herself in. Her mother would still be working at the supermarket checkout. With the longer hours that the store was now open she was seeing less of her mum than ever. She began the long wait for the letter from the Beacon by herself.

It was after nine when her mother got in. She just picked at the meal Gemma had made for her. "Oh, Mum," Gemma cried. "What is the point of you working such long hours if you come home exhausted?"

"That's what they want Gem, and you know it's about the only job I could get round here. So if they tell me they need me to work the extra hours, I've not got a lot of choice."

"But, Mum, you're worn out." Gemma hated her mother looking so tired. "You're not even forty and you look old."

Her mother almost laughed "I *feel* old. Tell me about the job you went for today."

Gemma told her, and her mother could feel the hope, the excitement inside of her daughter, and wished for her that she would not be disappointed.

Chapter Two

Entering The Beacon

Because they didn't have a phone, Gemma knew she would have to wait for a letter. So, each morning, she'd run downstairs when she saw the postman.

Three days after her interview, she was looking out of her window when she saw Barbara coming bustling down the alley, obviously checking the house numbers. Gemma went down, opened the cottage door and called to her. Barbara held out an envelope. "Mrs O'Halloran thought you'd like to know as soon as possible." Gemma really wanted to go inside, so she was by herself, just in case she hadn't got the job, but she didn't want to appear rude and anyway, Barbara was grinning. "Aren't you going to open it?" Gemma laughed. "You know what's in it, don't you?"

Gemma tore it open with her fingers. "Dear Gemma, I am very pleased…" Her eyes filled with tears of hope that hadn't been disappointed.

"I hope you'll enjoy working with us," said Barbara and she gave her a hug of congratulations.

Gemma soon learnt the ways of the Beacon. The residents got up when they wanted and made their own breakfast, which they ate in the dining area. Mid-morning was the daily meeting, where any problems in the unit – between residents or between staff and residents – could be aired, news exchanged and plans for the future made. Everyone – staff included – was expected to be there, unless it had been agreed otherwise in the meeting; so Beatrice and Tom came in from the beach.

Some of the residents spoke more than others. Mrs Austin said very little, and sometimes, when Tom spoke, he would get confused about when events happened. He'd talk as if events that happened years ago – like his brother dying – happened yesterday.

Mrs O'Halloran saw all the staff by themselves for an hour a week for supervision. In one of her first sessions, Gemma said she wasn't sure whether residents like Mrs Austin or Tom got much out of the meetings. Mrs O'Halloran told her that both had come with a diagnosis of dementia. "Some specialists say that dementia is a disease, which causes brain damage and memory problems. They say it's incurable. But I think we can help them get a bit better as long as we have enough staff who believe in their work, and if we don't take too many very confused residents. If they are in the majority, everyone – confused, or non-confused, resident or staff – descends into a hopeless craziness. But if the confused are in a minority, the other residents set the tone and can lift the one or two forgetful ones. So, yes, we can help Mrs Austin and Tom. What's vital is that we respect them and don't leave them out of decision-making. So, *they* must be included in the meetings, and then given the help they need to participate. You'll find the other residents understand this and do try to help them."

After that supervision session, Gemma started paying more attention to how residents helped each other in the meeting – by suggesting the words that another resident wanted to use but couldn't find; or supporting residents if they became scared that they were being too critical of staff. She also learnt how staff could encourage residents – by waiting for them to find the words; welcoming their contributions, however short, and showing an interest in what they said. She was impressed how Rose, in her motherly way, and how Barbara, with her "let's sort things out" manner, encouraged residents to voice their thoughts, sometimes just picking up on an unhappy look. Gemma also learnt that it was really important that staff members did not blindly defend and support each other; and that often, in fact, the residents were right in their complaints or worries.

Only Nurse Thompson didn't seem to find the meetings useful. She sat there because she had to, under sufferance, upright in her neatly ironed and starched uniform. It was nothing she said, but the way she sat and looked. Gemma felt a bit scared of her.

When Mrs O'Halloran had talked to her about confused behaviour, she had told her that a good working rule was "publicly acceptable behaviour in public places". Gemma saw this in action at lunchtime. Beatrice would occasionally try to eat food with her hands. One of Gemma's jobs was to remind her not to do this, by gently touching her arm, if she attempted to pick food with her fingers. Beatrice would give a little guilty laugh and usually pick up her knife and fork. Gemma quite enjoyed this task, partly because it seemed to be effective, and partly because Beatrice's fingers were long and beautiful.

In fact, mealtimes were one of the few times Beatrice – Mrs Hendry's first name and what she told Gemma she wanted her to call her by – was in the unit. She spent almost all her time at the east end of the beach, looking out over the water. She didn't say much and then only in single words or short sentences. Most often, she'd whisper "Dan, I do miss you", or "Dan, why did you have to go?". Dan was the name of her dead husband. Beatrice had outlived all her brothers and sisters as well as most of her friends. When she'd come in she had been dreadfully thin because she had neglected herself and her house had been in a terrible state.

Tom Dalgetty, who also spent most of his time outside, had been a fisherman – and he looked the part, with his thin, wiry body and strong arms, usually inside a navy-blue Guernsey pullover. His friends from the fishing boats still came to visit him, especially in the early evening when the bar in the Lookout was open. While Beatrice didn't move much on the foreshore, Tom was forever moving up and down and along the sand, beachcombing. Once he had registered that Gemma was at the Beacon to stay, he took to her and started calling her "Maid Gemma", and would bring her shells, rocks with fronds of dried seaweed, or pieces of dry, whitened wood twisted into strange shapes.

Of course, having two residents out of doors and at risk from the sea worried the staff but they respected their wishes. So both wore life-jackets over their clothes or coat when they went out. The life-jackets would inflate automatically if they fell into the sea. One staff member on each rota had the responsibility of checking where they were every ten minutes. This wasn't difficult. A security camera scanned the beach continuously, so Gemma only had to walk to the office and check the video display unit.

The last resident Gemma got to know was Mrs Tremayne. At first glance, there was nothing obviously wrong with her, but Gemma soon learnt what Mrs Tremayne's problem was – she wouldn't eat. At the table, she'd just push her food around the plate; often she refused to leave her room or the lounge area when told lunch was ready.

A few weeks after she had started, Gemma was working with Nurse Thompson on the morning shift. It was coming up to lunchtime. Tom had wandered in, so she went to get Beatrice off the beach.

As she came in, she could hear Mrs Tremayne complaining. She and Beatrice were overtaken by Mrs O'Halloran. They were just behind her as Mrs O'Halloran opened the door. Mrs Tremayne was in her chair and Nurse Thompson was leaning over her and pulling her by the wrists. "You *will* come and eat your lunch," she was shouting angrily.

"Nurse Thompson," called Mrs O'Halloran softly. The nurse whirled round – she hadn't heard Mrs O'Halloran come in. "Please come with me." Nurse Thompson walked to the door of the unit. She stopped in front of the Matron and glared at her in blank defiance. "Please get your coat and leave," said Mrs O'Halloran.

Beatrice and Gemma were rooted just behind Mrs O'Halloran and the nurse; and like all the residents, they watched to see what would happen.

"We will pay you a month's salary. Now please leave."

Nurse Thompson's mouth opened. She did not seem to believe what she was being told. She looked at the Matron and saw that she meant what she had said.

"You," she said "*You* are sacking *me*. Well, let me tell you something. This place is a shambles. The residents do just as they like – there's no discipline." Her voice was rising and she started to shout. "There is not enough medication; there are not enough nurses, just local girls who don't know what they're doing." She dropped her voice into a tone of threatening menace. "And people need to know what's happening here. And I mean to tell them."

"Just go," said Mrs O'Halloran. Nurse Thompson went to the coathooks and grabbed her coat; she went to her locker, got out her bag and slammed the metal door shut. Calmer now, she turned to address Mrs O'Halloran. "You," she said, "are a disgrace to the profession." She turned and walked out.

There was a silence. Then Beatrice said, "It's sad when people quarrel." It was the longest sentence Gemma had heard her say. Gemma, shocked by the whole episode, could only nod in agreement.

Chapter Three

Adam's Message

On a bright and sunny morning a few days later, Gemma decided that rather than use the security video, she'd go out onto the beach to check that Tom and Beatrice were OK. Beatrice, as usual, was looking out over the sea. Tom was shuffling along the line of sand and dune to check on what the sea had thrown up on the last high tide.

As she came back in, Rose said, "Your young man rang. He asked if you were off duty this weekend and, when I said you were, he left a message. He wants you to meet him at the steps down from the pier head at midday Saturday."

Your young man! Adam and Gemma had been in the same class at school and had gone out together in their last year. After they left school, they'd been too busy with their summer jobs to meet much, and things had drifted till she'd met him a few days ago in Fishertown and told him where she was working.

"Right, thanks," she said to Rose "If those are my instructions, I'd better be there then."

The stone pierhead at Fishertown ran out into the sea and ended in a circular platform on which sat the harbour light. Its purpose was to break the waves coming up into the harbour. The steps down its side looked out to the sea, so it was hard to see what was coming downstream. Gemma was just beginning to wonder if Adam was going to show up, when a dinghy with tan sails slipped past in a blur, and then there was a wooshing and a rattling and the dinghy had spun round and was coming back towards the steps. "Quick, jump in," Adam was shouting as he guided the boat alongside, and he put out a hand to help her.

Gemma grabbed his hand and scrambled on board. "Sit in front of me and watch out for the boom." Gemma knew that the boom was the heavy pole that held down the bottom of the mainsail.

Adam gave a push against the pier steps to spin the boat round. He pulled on some ropes. The sail was pushed to the other side of the boat by the wind and Gemma ducked as the boom sped across, creaking above her head. The wind coming down the river filled up the sails and soon the boat was screaming out to sea, a white wave breaking along its bow.

"She's called *Periwinkle*," Adam shouted across to her.

"Where did you get her from?" Gemma called to him.

"An old fella down my street had her in his garden. He said we could have her if we promised to do her up. 'Course, she needed a lot doing, so Paul and I took it on between jobs." Paul had been in the same class as Gemma and Adam, and, like Adam, now worked as a builder's labourer when there was work.

Now that they were sailing, Gemma had time to look at the dinghy. It was made of wood and had been varnished so lovingly, she could almost see her reflection.

Adam sailed *Periwinkle* round the island that lies to the west of Fishertown. Gemma had been in a dinghy once or twice years ago, so it was not all totally new. She took the ropes that controlled the foresail, and soon was pulling it smoothly across from one side of the boat to the other when Adam moved the boat through the wind.

As they headed back into the river, along the pier wall, Adam asked, "When's the next time you're off?" Gemma told him that the weekend after next she'd be free from Saturday midday to Monday morning.

"Great, I'll meet you on Lantern Beach around midday Saturday. Bring some warm clothes and some food. We'll make a weekend of it."

He pulled up the boom, so that the mainsail folded, and the boat slowed. Gemma scrambled out onto the steps. Adam dropped the sail back down and *Periwinkle* started sailing again and then was lost to Gemma's sight as the boat rounded a bend in the river.

In the days that followed, Gemma got to understand two of the residents better – by taking Mrs Bennett to hospital, and the Corporal to church.

Mrs Bennett's outpatient appointments in the local hospital were at the oncology clinic. "That means cancer, dear," Mrs Bennett told her, in a matter-of-fact sort of way, the first time that Gemma accompanied her. Long waits to be seen and to have the tests gave plenty of time to talk, which sometimes Mrs Bennett wanted to do; sometimes she preferred silence. On one occasion she told Gemma, "The cancer was the reason I'd wanted to come to the Beacon. I'm a widow and our only child, my daughter, is in Australia. I wanted to face up to the cancer, if that's what I've definitely got, but I didn't want to do it alone."

Mr Dawson was called "Corporal" by the residents and staff alike. One of his favourite phrases was "Fought my way up from El Alamein to the coast of Africa and then up Italy," said in clipped tones, but not with a great deal of pride or contentment. Perhaps that was why he liked going to church. Mrs O'Halloran discouraged ministers – or hairdressers for that matter – from coming and performing their services in the home. Rather, she encouraged the residents to get out of the home to use their services, if they wanted to.

Gemma was working the next Sunday, so she was detailed to help the Corporal and, more specifically, George, to get to St Keverne, the church at the top of the hill that overlooked Lantern Beach.

George Meredith had been in the Navy and was more philosophical about the War. "Twelve Atlantic crossings from 1939 to 1942 when the U-boats controlled that ocean – lucky to be alive. Not many of my mates in those convoys are."

Like many of the residents, after the war he'd found work in Plymouth – the women worked as shop assistants or as domestics, the men in the dockyard. But if George had been lucky in the war, he had been less lucky in his peacetime job. He had chronic emphysema from the asbestos around the condensers he'd worked on as a boilerman. It was the emphysema that had damaged his lungs and made him so short of breath. So, one of the staff would drive him in the minibus to the church.

Usually it was Steve. He would come in even on his days off ("It's nae bother," he'd say in his Glaswegian accent) and drive them up. After the service, George could manage walking back down if they made enough stops.

For Gemma, this was the first time she had gone to church since she was at school. To hear hymns sung by people to whom they obviously meant a great deal; to sit beneath the semicircles of black rafters and hear the hymns and prayers and the sermon echo around – this was strange to her.

The Corporal did not sing or say his amens with any fervour. Being there seemed to be enough. As they walked back down the hill after the service, he would sometimes say things like "I made a mess of my life", but wouldn't explain to them what he meant.

Other staff had little more success in trying to understand why the war had been so damaging to the Corporal.

Besides attending the daily meetings, Mrs O'Halloran would come into the unit to help when her other work allowed. One morning, when they were sitting down over a coffee, Gemma decided to pick her brains as to how she could help unhappy people – she was thinking of the Corporal in particular.

"Well," said Mrs O'Halloran, putting her coffee cup down, "not just by giving them medication. Being very unhappy and not being able to see the reason for it is depression, but most older people are unhappy for a real reason. Maybe they made a wrong decision earlier in their lives and it's had serious consequences; perhaps they treated someone badly; or they've lost too many people they loved or too many things they valued – a few of our residents have quarrelled with their children and now don't know how to mend the fences. So they aren't sad without cause. They're unhappy for very good reasons. We can help them by encouraging them to talk about what's making them sad and helping them work out what they can do about it, and we can call in people to help us. Perhaps it's time I got Mrs Cooper, the psychotherapist, back to see if we should be doing more."

Chapter Four

Voyage to the Dodman

The following Saturday, Gemma packed a change of clothes and some food. As she went onto the beach just before midday, she saw *Periwinkle* in the bay. She went down to the waterline. Adam brought the boat ashore. They stowed Gemma's gear and she hopped aboard.

"A northwester," Adam said as they drew away from the shore. "Perfect for a run down to the Dodman." And *Periwinkle* seemed to agree – she positively flew across the wavelets down south by west towards the great headland.

In these calm conditions, Adam had the time to show Gemma how to helm the boat and how to know when the sails were happy and when they weren't drawing properly. So, to get the boat sailing well, she had to pull the sails tighter or looser by using the sheets – the ropes that controlled them. He also showed Gemma how you could feel where the wind was coming from by which bit of your neck felt cold, and by looking at the top of the mast where there was a wind arrow. She needed to keep checking where the wind was because the direction of the wind can change from one minute to the next and then she had to adjust the sails again to keep the boat's speed up.

At first, Gemma felt overwhelmed by all this information, all these things she could get wrong but, after a while, she started to get the hang of watching what was happening and responding appropriately.

After an hour or so, Adam relieved her of the helm, and she could relax. She watched Adam guiding the boat through the water. She realized that Adam did matter to her even though he was no whizz-kid. He wasn't terribly good-looking, although working outdoors had bleached his hair and had given him muscles he hadn't had when they were at school. But she trusted him, and trusted herself with him, to him – like now, when they were in the middle of nowhere.

In another hour, they were closing the Dodman, which reared above them like a great sleeping hound. There was a long, grey, gritty beach on its flank. Adam sailed *Periwinkle* into the shallow foam and then they carried her up over the tideline.

It was a steep climb to the top. As they gained height, there were no trees, only scrub bushes. The breeze felt colder, and the song of the birds in the hedgerows purer. Butterflies with large brown wings with red eyes painted on them flitted across their path. They reached the spine of the hill and there saw the large cross on the headland that the local vicar had long ago built for the souls of the sailors lost in the waters below.

They could see for miles. Behind them was a large embankment over which a couple of buzzards drifted lazily. The ancient Britons must have built it as a defence against invaders. Further to the north were the giant white spoil heaps of the china clay pits around St Austell; far to the east the triangle of Rame Head; up and down the channel, steamers and tankers pushed along on their journeys; and to the west, just the endless blue sea. "New York next stop," said Adam. He picked up a stone and threw it over the cliff edge and they heard it bounce down.

It was late afternoon by the time they got back to *Periwinkle* and set sail. The wind had dropped and Adam saw there was no hope of them getting back to Lantern Bay or even Fishertown in the light. "It's not safe to sail without lights in the dark – we could get run down by a fishing boat. We'll go up the coast as far as we can and then we'll run her ashore for the night." They made a few miles to the north. Already, Gemma could see the flashing light from the lighthouse at the end of a harbour wall. "Meva," said Adam as he started heading the boat inshore. "We'll be going ashore at Pentewan." Pentewan was one of the harbours built to export the china clay from the pits around St Austell, but which had fallen into disuse. In a little while they were pulling the boat up the beach into the harbour channel, now completely covered by sand. Once they had sorted out the sails, they walked up the channel inside the ruins of the long quay wall till they came to the old lock gates that kept in the water of the harbour.

In the village they bought some fish and chips and ate them on the old harbour wall. By the time they made their way back to the boat it was getting dark. It was too early in the season for holidaymakers so the beach was theirs alone. There was plenty of wood brought in on the high tide and then marooned in the entrance channel. They gathered large armfuls and heaped it up. Using some old paper that had blown onto the beach, Adam had no difficulty getting a fire started and, as they sat close to its blazing heat and light, Adam told her about his uncle who had worked in the claypits in the country behind them. His uncle had spent most time in one of the largest and deepest pits – Half Mile Pit – and Adam told of how he had seen him washing out the creamy white clay with high-powered hoses and then getting it pumped away to be dried. Gemma felt at peace as she listened to Adam's story and watched the fire through closing eyes, and heard its crackling behind and between Adam's words.

Eventually the fire burnt down and they sat in a silence complete except for the rhythm of the waves as they broke gently on the beach. It was a clear night and the sky was a black screen with a thousand stars on it. Adam pointed out Venus and Orion and the saucepan shape of the guide stars for the Pole Star. "It always tells you where the north is. What do you think is underneath it?"

Gemma looked at the Pole Star and considered. "Lostwithiel?" she answered hesitatingly. Adam laughed.

Without the fire, it was getting cold and Adam got a groundsheet and a blanket out of the locker in the dinghy and they lay down to sleep. Adam fell asleep with his arm across his face. Before dawn, while the night was still black, he started stirring restlessly and mumbling in his sleep. "The pit. Must get out… Can't grasp the sides. Everything white and smooth…it's all crumbling… No-one there to help. No escape." Gemma nudged him awake and then she held him to her till he settled and fell asleep until the sun rose high enough for its beams to burn through their eyelids.

They woke while the rest of the world was still asleep. There was only one man from the caravan site, walking his dog. They got some fresh water from the village and boiled up a saucepan for tea. Adam held the cup between his hands and stared out at the turquoise sea. He flicked his hair out of his eyes, which Gemma knew he did when he was nervous. "Gem," he said, "you know there's no decent work for me in Fishertown. Would you leave here? Could we go away together up-country?"

She could only answer, "I couldn't leave the Beacon – not now – not yet."

Chapter Five

After Pentewan

It was the birds that told Gemma that summer was coming – the quick flitting terns on the shore, the swallows swooping for flies low over the dunes.

But the coming of summer did not cheer Adam up. If anything, it made him more moody. Gemma was afraid that he was upset by her reply on Pentewan beach. One Friday night, they went out for a drink and a meal in Fishertown. They spent more than she could afford and Adam drank quite a lot. When they came out of the restaurant Gemma realized it must be late. The town was quiet – she couldn't hear the hum of the fridges and the generators of the cafés; and the smell of chips and pasties no longer clung to the air. They walked along the fishermen's quay, where the catches were unloaded. The boats tied up alongside were bobbing quietly in the night breeze, the smell of fishmeal heavy on the night air. The drink had cheered Adam at first and put him in good humour. But now, as the reflected street lights flickered in the black water, there was no peace in him. He was filled with discontent – his building work was irregular and the pay was low. "A good night out like tonight and you practically blow a week's wages," he said angrily. "I could be earning double in London." The trouble was that Gemma knew that what he was saying was true, and she couldn't help him or change things for him.

Now, she stood outside the Beacon, waiting for him. She could smell the sea carried on a chill wind and the odour of the seaweed wrack broken off and brought in on the tide. She pulled her jumper around her. There was a dot out to sea. Suddenly she realized it was *Periwinkle* and it was heading into Lantern Beach. Soon Adam was ashore and kissing her.

"What are you doing?" she asked, for he'd made no mention of going sailing.

"Today's the day. We're leaving."

Gemma was caught by surprise. Of course she knew he was fed up and wanted to leave Fishertown. "But how… But why?"

"Paul says he's got a mate who can get us loads of work up in London."

"But Adam, how are you going to get there? It's an awfully long way in *Periwinkle*; will you be safe?"

He laughed and held a hand to his ear in mock attention. So she listened too; and from behind the dunes she could hear an engine getting louder; and as it got more distinct, she recognized it as the engine of a motorcycle;

and then it came round the final bend – a black, powerful motorcycle and Paul was riding it.

Adam was exultant. "Paul's dad had had it in his garage for ages; it's an old Triumph. It was always going to be our next project after *Periwinkle.*"

Paul drew the bike up alongside the two. "I'm sorry it's this ugly hulk and not you, Gem," Adam said, "but I've got to give it a try – the chance may not come again." It was as if he wanted her permission.

She looked at the two of them. They were so young. London was so far away. Why did they have to go?

There was a silence that none of them seemed able to break. *Periwinkle*'s sails flapped on the breeze. "What will happen to her?" asked Gemma. Adam walked over to *Periwinkle* and ran his hand along her finely varnished side. "She's a present to you from Paul and me. We want you to have her. We've left you our buoyancy aids, and we've even put an extra strip on the keel so you won't hurt her if you're by yourself and you have to drag her up the beach."

Adam took his helmet from Paul. "Hoi, you, on the pillion," he said. "I'm driving this thing till I see the Tamar beneath me. Then you can ride her to hell and back." He turned to Gemma and held her to him, kissing her long and hard.

He looked directly into her eyes. "Next time I come back, it'll be to take you with me. That's a promise." Then he jumped on the bike, kicked it into life, engaged the gears and roared off along the beach. She heard it whining up over the dunes and the duller thud of the engine as it climbed the hill, and then only its echo reverberated to her. She waited till she could no longer hear any sound of the machine. Gemma held back her tears. She could have gone with him, but that meant leaving the Beacon and she couldn't do that. Now she just felt deserted as if, for all his promises, she'd never see Adam again.

She became aware of Tom standing near her.

"Is she yours now, Maid Gemma?" he said, pointing at the boat. She nodded. "Well, we'll have to do what the lad asked and look after her. Let's get her safely up the beach and get her gear stowed."

Chapter Six

A Trip to Fishertown

The arrival of *Periwinkle* seemed to give Tom new purpose. Now, whenever Gemma had any spare time, he wanted to teach her how to sail the boat properly – how to work out whether the tide was ebbing or flooding by whether the sand below the tide line was wet or dry; how to look at the sky and the clouds to see what the weather had in store; how to launch the dinghy when the wind was coming from various directions. Sometimes he couldn't find the words, and he'd curse in frustration when he couldn't hand on his fisherman's experience, but usually Gemma could work out what he wanted to say, and would check it out. If she got it right, Tom would beam at her.

Mrs O'Halloran and Gemma had discussed Tom taking her to sea and the safety of both Tom and herself in the dinghy. "From what you tell me," Mrs O'Halloran concluded, "it sounds like he knows what he's doing and he's using old skills that he obviously hasn't forgotten. As long as you feel good, sail with him." Gemma always did feel good and safe and over the next few weeks, with Tom's tuition, she became quite skilled at handling *Periwinkle*.

One morning, Tom came into Mrs O'Halloran's office and, pointing to the cloudless, blue sky, said he wanted to make a longer sail with Gemma – to Fishertown. When Mrs O'Halloran, after seeing Gemma was in agreement, gave her permission, Tom said he needed some money, but didn't or couldn't say why. Because Tom had some time ago lost his understanding of the value of money, the home was the guardian of his finances and kept his pension for him. Mrs O'Halloran was happy for him to take out twenty pounds – it was his money and he could do what he wanted with it. After lunch, Tom and Gemma went out to the beach, put on their buoyancy aids, and got the dinghy down to the surfline and there they hoisted sail and were soon heading west.

The breeze was from the west. A sailing boat cannot sail into the wind, so they had to first tack one side of the wind and then the other. But it was not too far, so soon they could make the river inside the pierhead and, pushed in by the first of the flood tide, sailed up river till they could tie up alongside a crabber. The skipper needed another two hours of water before he could get across the bar, so didn't mind them leaving *Periwinkle* tied onto his boat as long as they were back in time.

Once ashore, although he had not been in Fisher-town for a long time, Tom had no difficulty orientating himself. He hurried along the quay till he reached the ferry steps. The little ferry chugged across the river and landed them at the fish quay. Tom obviously remembered the old town and its alleys well and strode along so fast that Gemma had trouble keeping up. A number of people recognized and greeted him, but he only spoke to them briefly. Gemma guessed he'd forgotten their names and that he was worried he'd lose the thread of the conversation. Perhaps he was scared he might forget what was on the list in his head.

He hurried on to the chandlers and started looking at the mackerel lines. He held them and looked at the feathers attentively, before making his selection. Then, with equal care, he looked for a knife. He made the assistant open the display so that he could check the quality of each knife's steel and its sharpness on his thumb. Eventually, to the evident relief of the impatient assistant, he made his selection. He held out his money to the cashier, and Gemma checked his change for him.

Once out of the shop, they were nearly back where *Periwinkle* was moored when Tom suddenly changed direction and headed off for a tobacconist and bought a box of matches. Then, he picked up the first newspaper he saw and bought that too.

Only now that his purchases were complete did Tom relax. "Used to be fishing boats coming in under sail when I was a nipper; and if they couldn't sail in, I'd help pull them in from the harbour entrance up to the quay. The skipper would let you take a few fish as thanks. And when the herring were running, there'd be so many fishing boats working that if the weather was bad and they had to stay in port, you could practically cross the river on them."

By the time they had sailed clear of the harbour mouth, the tide was flooding up-channel, which was their direction home. Tom sailed *Periwinkle* out into the bay and kept looking all around. He pointed to a small flock of gannets. The large, sleek white birds with yellow faces and black wing tips were wheeling around a patch of water and then one would plummet and dive-bomb head first into the water for a fish it had seen. "There'll be mackerel under them," said Tom and he headed *Periwinkle* out towards the flock. As he neared, he reduced the size of the mainsail, so they were sailing very slowly – "Just on the tide," he said – and then he ran his mackerel line with its coloured feathers out from the back of the boat.

They sailed in silence for a few minutes, the only activity being Tom hauling his line in towards him, feeling its weight and then letting it go again. Suddenly the line went taut. Tom carefully grasped it and pulled it slowly towards him. Gemma could now see a flash of silver as the fish tried to pull away from the hook, but Tom kept reeling it in till it was by the boat. Then he pulled it up and into the boat; and, quickly grasping the fish by its body, he banged its head on the side of the cockpit with two quick thwacks, and put the fish into the well of the boat where it lay still. "You must put them out of their misery," he said, looking at Gemma, "and not let them suffocate."

In this way, Tom caught three more mackerel. Two came up together. After he had caught these four, he brought his line in. "Four is enough. Only catch what you can use." He wound the line away, carefully embedding the hooks in the lines. "A cork is even better," he said. The line safely coiled, they hoisted sail and Gemma steered for Lantern Bay. Meanwhile, Tom got out his newly acquired knife and picked up the first fish. He cut it open along the underneath of its belly and then, with his finger, drew out the entrails and threw them in the sea. The seagulls soon saw what he was doing and a small flock quickly gathered to dive, fight, and squabble noisily over each further offering. When he had gutted all the fish, he leant over the side and washed each one, making the water bloody. By this time, Gemma had reached Lantern Beach and was running the boat ashore. After the gear was stowed, Tom told her to find small pieces of driftwood. "Dry wood," he said, "as dry as you can get."

Once Gemma started looking, she quickly found many pieces that the spring tides had deposited high up the beach and, in a few minutes, had a small pile of whitened wood. Tom took the unread newspaper, and laid a few pages out fully, and then he rolled up the rest into little balls which he placed over the sheets. Then came the small pieces of wood. He lit the fire which soon burnt fiercely. "Stones?" he asked Gemma. She brought him some and he placed them on each side of the now fiercely glowing embers. He took one of the fish and spread it open either side of its spine; then he placed the fish on the stones across the fire. As the fish cooked, fat dropped onto the fire, feeding it and keeping it hot, and soon Tom gave Gemma a cooked mackerel steak.

From his jacket pocket, he took out a twist of newspaper. He opened it and there were grains of pepper. He put some on her steak. Then, delving again inside his jacket, he produced two slightly battered slices of bread. Gemma was surprised at the planning that he must have done – planning done by a man who literally did not know the time of day. "Next time we'll take a piece of lemon – it'll make it even better," he said. Gemma, her mouth full of freshly cooked fish, its juices running down the side of her mouth, wanted to laugh with pleasure at the taste, but could only nod carefully in agreement.

Chapter Seven

Return to Rame

Gemma gradually got to know the specialist staff who came in for sessions at the Beacon. Brenda, the physio, ran regular keep-fit classes for residents and staff, and also helped with any problems clients had in using their arms and legs. Kathy, the occupational therapist, took it as a personal challenge to make the preparation of the meals by the residents a reality – not them standing by, watching the staff. She aimed to make cooking achievable for everyone, no matter how immobile or even wheelchair bound they might be or how twisted their hands might have become from arthritis or a stroke. She did this by raising or lowering surfaces, fixing supports, buying or even designing special cutlery and implements.

For those who had forgotten what they were supposed to be doing, her motto was "Small steps, help when needed, and no failures." She saw Mrs Austin as a particular challenge. Gemma had come to recognize that even the simplest task seemed to overwhelm Mrs Austin so that she either made mistakes or dithered around, paralysed by her confusion. Gemma liked to watch Kathy at work, breaking every task down into steps and helping the person achieve them – like the morning Mrs Austin came to breakfast in her usual state of uncertainty. Kathy almost seemed to pounce on her. "Mrs Austin, what tickles your palate today?"

Mrs Austin gazed at her, slightly bewildered. "An egg," she said. "Yes, a boiled egg."

"And a boiled egg you shall have." Kathy knelt down beside her. "Where are the eggs?"

Mrs Austin looked helplessly around the room. Then she noticed that Kathy was staring at the fridge so, hesitatingly, she pointed at the fridge.

"Great," said Kathy. "Better check that the gannets have left you one."

Mrs Austin walked across to the fridge and opened it. There was a row of eggs. She took one out.

"Right, something to boil it in?"

Mrs Austin reached for a saucepan that was hanging up nearby and then, without any prompting, filled it with water from the tap.

"Marvellous," said Kathy. "Would you like Gemma to help you light the gas?"

Mrs Austin had bad arthritis in her hands, so lighting the gas was very difficult for her. She agreed. Gemma lit the gas and Mrs Austin put the pan on the stove.

"How long do you reckon it will take to boil the egg? Three minutes? Five minutes?"

Mrs Austin thought five minutes was about right. Kathy set the timer for five minutes and they buttered some bread whilst they waited. When the alarm sounded, Mrs Austin took a large scoop with a rubber handle and fished the egg out and, with a bit of wheedling, she got it in the egg cup. She sat down, bashed the top and pushed it off with her spoon. Then she looked round for the salt and shook some onto the egg, and then broke into a smile of delight as she tasted her first mouthful. "Really good," she declared.

Mrs Cooper, the psychotherapist, was also now coming regularly. She was a quiet-spoken, middle-aged lady, well-dressed, slightly formal and old-fashioned. The Corporal, rather to the staff's surprise, had agreed to see her; and, having had one session, now saw her weekly.

The staff had suggested to Beatrice that she might like to see Mrs Cooper but she had refused. When they persisted she'd just say, "Dan's all I've got left."

Mrs Cooper had also been asked to help those residents the staff were having difficulty with. One of these was Mrs Tremayne, who was still very picky and uncooperative at mealtimes. Mrs Cooper spent some time with her and then, with the staff including Gemma. She listened far more than she spoke.

It turned out that no-one really knew much about Martha Tremayne. She had come in late one Friday, having neglected herself at home. Shortly after that, her social worker went off on long-term sick leave for stress, and the promised background information had never arrived, despite the Beacon asking for it on several occasions.

Martha had no relatives to fill in the gaps. She had lived in a small village on the Rame peninsula. Mrs Cooper suggested that it might help jog her memory if she went back there with a member of staff to see if together they could find out more about her life. Gemma volunteered to go with her and felt pleased when Mr Mitchell, with some difficulty, wished them well and the other residents joined in with those good wishes.

They took the Plymouth bus that went across the Tamar on the ferry. It was a slow journey east as the bus detoured to take in every holiday camp and every cluster of chalets. Gemma passed the time listening to the conversations of the housewives planning their shopping trips in the city centre.

At last they arrived at a small village green, next to a church with a stubby spire, and got off. Gemma's plan was to walk to Mrs Tremayne's old house to see if neighbours would recognize her and talk about old times, and then, perhaps, try the local shop or the pub.

Gemma had the address but there was no need to ask anyone the way; Mrs Tremayne was quite clear where her old home was and they soon reached the cottage – but there was no-one there. Judging by the furnishings that Gemma could see through the window, she thought it had become a holiday home.

Nor did any neighbours conveniently pop out to greet Mrs Tremayne. But as they walked up to the village centre, they were stopped by a young man in his thirties. He looked puzzled as if he knew Mrs Tremayne but wasn't quite sure. "It is – it isn't – you are Mrs Tremayne, aren't you?" She was pleased at the recognition. "Mrs Tremayne – my old primary school teacher."

"And you're Robert Roundle," Mrs Tremayne said. Gemma was amazed. In the Beacon Mrs Tremayne didn't say very much. On the occasions she spoke, it was usually to the floor or her plate.

Mrs Tremayne and Robert Roundle were soon talking like long-lost friends. True, the younger man did much of the talking, and most of the reminiscing, but Mrs Tremayne clearly remembered the events he recalled of his days at the village school, and even added a few details.

It turned out that, besides her lessons, Mrs Tremayne had also taught music. "You played the piano at assembly every morning." Mrs Tremayne smiled modestly. "Of course," he said to Gemma, "the school shut down years ago."

He turned back to Mrs Tremayne. "I've got a confession to make. When I heard that up-country people had bought your place and all the fittings after you left so suddenly – well, I couldn't bear for them to have your cello, because you used to play it on special occasions in the school. You'd never tell us when, as it was supposed to be a surprise for us, but *I* knew because I'd hear you rehearsing in your cottage after school. Well, when I heard about the sale and that some London solicitor was going to get your cello, I'm afraid I got in one night and took it, so that he shouldn't have it. Of course, it wasn't any good to me 'cos I didn't know how to even get a note out of the beast. So I put it in the loft – at least there it was safe. But – oh, it's so good to see you – of course you must have it back."

There was no arguing with him. He insisted on them coming back to his house to reclaim it and, not without difficulty, he got the cello in its case down from the attic. There was still more than an hour left before the bus home arrived, so he made them both a cup of tea and got out the biscuits. Gemma noticed that in these surroundings Mrs Tremayne's table manners were impeccable, taking little mouthfuls of biscuit, and holding the saucer while she drank – even holding her little finger crooked! She and Mr Roundle went on talking about the old times, and Gemma watched as Mrs Tremayne changed from being a listener to a storyteller, talking about the village and village life – changed from being a woman without a past to the well-respected school teacher with her husband, the village carpenter; and the mother of a daughter living somewhere in Plymouth; and, of course, a superb cello player.

As the time came to get their bus, he escorted them to the bus stop, carrying the cello. Gemma said a silent prayer that the bus would not be full. It wasn't, and the bus driver seemed to think it rather amusing to see a cello in his luggage compartment.

When they got off, they walked to the nearest phone box and leant the cello against it. Gemma rang to be picked up in a car big enough to take both the cello and them back to the Beacon.

Fortunately, Steve was on and he brought the van up; and soon the cello was once more reunited with Mrs Tremayne in her room.

Chapter Eight

Summer Nights

With the coming of summer, life moved outside. The residents spent much more time on the beach, sunning themselves in deckchairs. They would bring lunch out and arrange it on trestle tables. An adventurous few – like George and Mrs Bennett – even had a bit of a swim.

For Gemma, Adam's gift of *Periwinkle* changed her life that summer. Now in the evenings, after she finished work, she would go sailing. In the beginning, she usually took Tom so that he could teach her but, as the summer days became longer, increasingly she felt confident enough to take *Periwinkle* out by herself, especially at weekends, for greater distances. She returned to Pentewan, and remembered her trip there with Adam. They had kept in touch, and London was suiting him well. He was earning good money, and in his phone calls to her, he told of fantastic clubs and gigs he'd been to.

Mrs O'Halloran knew of Gemma's changing life, if only because Gemma was keeping more of her things at the Beacon. In one of their supervision sessions, Mrs O'Halloran told her that she did not object, but she hoped that Gemma would keep in touch with her mother. Gemma promised her she would.

She could now catch and cook mackerel, thanks to Tom. And Tom gave her another gift. A large stone with a hole in it – a sharpening stone wheel – had been washed up on the beach by a gale. A couple of days later, he found a long piece of rope. He showed it to Gemma with delight. She sat on a rock and watched as he put the rope through the hole in the stone and then separated the strands of the rope. He bent them over the stone and back into the rope. "It's an eye splice, Maid Gemma," he explained. He tested it for strength and, when he was satisfied, took out his knife and cut the loose ends neatly away. "There's your anchor, my maid, but only for calm nights."

So now, with fine weather, she no longer needed to cycle home when she finished work. Instead, she would prepare the dinghy, launch it and sail it out in the light breeze, away over the turquoise sea. Letting the sails flap, she'd stop the boat and lose the sweat of a hot day's work by slipping over the side into the cooling water. Diving down, scaring shoals of small fish that darted away, deep towards the golden seabed with its plants and shells, she would feel the water sliding across her hair, her face, her whole body, till she had to return, gasping, to the surface. She would cling to the side of *Periwinkle*, taking great gulps of air into her starved lungs; and then, when she felt ready, she would submerge herself again and return to the blue deep where there was only herself, and her strong young body carving its way through the infinity of water.

When she was satisfied, she would lie on a towel along the inside of *Periwinkle*, letting her body dry in the rays of the evening sun. Sometimes she fished for mackerel, but usually she packed herself some food. She would eat it out on the deep water before sailing inshore and letting go the anchor stone; and then, tucking herself into her sleeping bag with a topsheet to keep off the morning dew, she would settle down for the night. Occasionally, a seabird would startle her by flying into *Periwinkle*'s rigging before disentangling itself, or a cormorant would fly rapidly by her as it powered its black body along the waves, looking for a good place to find food.

As she went to sleep, she would see the beam flashing from the lighthouse guarding the Eddystone reefs. Later in the night, if it became a bit windy and the waves began to rock the boat, a quick glance would tell her if she was on the same line as when she went to sleep. Besides, if the anchor dragged and she drifted too near the shore, the sound of the breaking surf quickly roused her.

But such alarms were rare. Most usually she slept through till the cold of the dawn chilled her into wakefulness and she would rise to see the mist covering the hills above the sea. Sometimes, more strangely, it hid the sea, making the cliffs and headlands look like sea serpents wriggling and moving on their way out to the deep.

Then she would sail or row the dinghy onto the beach. When she had tidied *Periwinkle* away, she would go indoors for breakfast, for she found that after a night at sea she was always ravenously hungry.

The nights when she could escape in *Periwinkle* became very precious to Gemma, a secret no-one else could share; and she felt different – purer and more complete – out there drifting in the tide and sleeping below the stars.

Chapter Nine

Midsummer Night

At one of the house meetings in May, Mrs O'Halloran said that she had had a letter from the students of the Fourth Age.

"Some of you will remember them from last year. Anyway, they're a bunch of eighty year olds – in fact you've got to be eighty or older to join – that's why they say they're in their Fourth Age – and they like to study and have fun together. They've been coming here for a few years now. They write each year asking for permission to camp on the lawn, and use our facilities for their classes. In the past, we've always said yes, provided all their classes are open to our residents, and they organise a Midsummer Night's concert."

The residents were happy to give their permission. "Liven the place up, they do," said Mr Mitchell.

"The concert was lovely," said Mrs Austin.

Once it had been agreed, Mrs O'Halloran had a word with Gemma. "They're pretty self-sufficient, but we want to be helpful, so I'd like you to work with them in the daytime. In the evenings, they'll be doing their cooking and getting themselves to the pub."

Within a few days, the lawn disappeared: first with the arrival of two Portakabins for use as classrooms and for rehearsal space for the concert; and then with the arrival of the students themselves, who set up their tents and cooking areas.

A day later, their classes started. Each day started with a keep-fit half hour. Brenda, the physio, had agreed to run it and, in fact, the exercises were much the same as the voluntary morning keep-fit that the Beacon ran. The funny thing was that residents who made excuses or refused point-blank to attend the in-house activity were keen to attend the same one when it was run for the students.

There was a variety of academic and practical classes. One of them was figure drawing. Gemma, as usual, was around in the background as the students sketched the nude male model posing slightly uncomfortably in the middle of a Portakabin classroom. "The trouble is," she overheard one of the students say to another, "his fiddly bits – Harold always undressed in the dark, so I very rarely got to see his fiddly bits."

"Well then, you'll have to draw them from feeling, won't you, dear? Anyway, if you line them up with the window edge, at least they'll stay still."

The students certainly seemed to enjoy themselves, and their classes gave the residents a buzz. Gemma saw this when she ran the bar in the Lookout. In the long summer evenings, most of the residents would come up to watch the blood-red orange sun going down over the darkened sea.

The Corporal and George were talking. "Reminds me of Plymouth before D-day," said George. "Loads of people arriving, stacks of equipment – I was just terrified Gerry would get wind of it and start bombing us again."

"They certainly brighten the place up," said the Corporal. "And it'll get even more hectic as they get nearer the concert. I envy them – they're about the same age as us. It makes you think."

"Well, perhaps we should do something for the concert. We can use their rehearsal rooms."

"Well, why not?"

Mrs Tremayne also caught the mood, for she asked Gemma to help her find new strings for her cello and some rosin for her bow.

The concert was to take place in the open space next to the Beacon. Gemma worked with the students whilst they cleared the area, took delivery of some flooring and laid it down to make a dance-floor area. She worried as they put up the bandstand and the refreshment tent. She tried to do the bits that required standing on chairs and ladders, but her offers were usually politely and firmly refused by the students.

As for what would happen on the night, that was a secret. Anyone could ask to perform but they had to show they had some ability. Gemma was pretty certain that the Corporal and George were planning something and that they'd even roped Steve in somehow, but every time she asked one of them, she would only get winks or they would tap their noses with their fingers. She found them infuriating.

Everyone involved could invite relatives or friends to the concert. On a trip back home, Gemma asked her mother to come. She wanted her to see where she worked, to meet the people of the Beacon community, for that was how she now felt about her workplace, but her mother couldn't be persuaded. She wasn't sure she could get the time off work but, even more, she didn't want to intrude on Gemma's new life. "It wouldn't be right Gem – I'd be out of place and just get in your way." And no argument, no pleading on Gemma's part, could make her change her mind.

It was such a long night that afterwards Gemma couldn't remember everything that happened. She spent much of the time with Mrs Bennett, partly because Mrs Bennett seemed to be getting slower and frailer, and partly because this way she could have a guide to what was happening.

The concert did not start till it got dark. Before then, there was food and drink – although little drink was consumed – and a disco playing old music, which didn't attract a great deal of interest.

There were a number of acts after that – Gemma could vaguely recall a juggler, a tenor and a magician.

After an interval, the lights went off and a spotlight came on. From the band area came a drum roll. The members of the band walked on with their instruments and took a bow in the spotlight. The audience clapped and whistled in anticipation. Then, just as the lights came back up, the band launched into its first number. "This'll get them going," said Mrs Bennett. "Nothing like a swing band to get people on their feet."

And it did. Almost from the first note, people started asking each other for a dance and couples were going onto the dance floor. Mobility was no problem – people held those who needed support; others danced with a person in a wheelchair to the beat of the music; and quite a few of the pairs were two women. "*Moonlight Serenade*," explained Mrs Bennett. "Glen Miller's signature tune – a very, very popular band in the war. Of course, girls had to dance together as the men were away fighting. That was until the GIs, the American soldiers, came," she chuckled at her memories "which caused no end of troubles."

The whole place was jumping now and the dancing became frenetic. One tune had lots of false endings and then a big crescendo at the end. "*In the Mood...* I always thought the false endings were to give the couples that were canoodling time to adjust their dress," Mrs Bennett said with a laugh. Tune followed tune. A female singer – one of the students – joined the band and her renditions received great applause.

Then the lights on the bandstand went out. The lights on the dance-floor were also switched off. For a minute there was silence – the audience was resentful at this break in their enjoyment. But nothing happened, and they fell silent. The only light came from the moon, which had risen out of the sea. Out of the silence, from far down the beach, thin music could be heard dimly. Two men in black suits were walking slowly along the beach playing a penny-whistle and a mouth-organ and, a little distance behind, a third man was softly tapping out a death-march beat on a snare drum. Gemma looked at Mrs Bennett. "It's the theme from *The Bridge on the River Kwai*, about the war with Japan." Slowly the music came nearer. The audience was very still. Gemma could see the men in the moonlight. They were the Corporal and George, with Steve behind them. It must be costing George a lot to do this, she thought – and then she could see the Corporal clearly in the moonlight. Tears were streaming down his face. They kept walking and slowly the music faded. The audience stood very quietly.

After a short while, the band started up again. A woman with flounced skirts and many petticoats was doing a complicated dance with a man in a suit and bow tie. Everyone seemed more animated, the dancing more urgent and frenetic. "Jitterbugging was always like that," Mrs Bennett said. "The worse the air-raid, the more furiously they danced the next evening." The band played on.

At last people started drifting away. Gemma went into the Beacon and had cocoa with the staff and residents who were still up. Her head was full of the music she had heard and her eyes still full of the dancing she had seen. She went outside for a last look. In a couple of hours, the dawn would be breaking over the now silent landscape, but now the night was getting darker as the moon set. She gave a wide yawn, rubbed her eyes and went back indoors.

Chapter Ten

Aftermath

Everyone slept late the next morning and most of the residents started their day with an early lunch. The afternoon passed quietly and then, as if by some unwritten agreement, they all went up to the Lookout. Gemma, too, had slept in. She came on for the evening shift and was behind the bar.

Everyone was saying how much they had enjoyed the previous evening and how it had brought back lots of memories. Many of them were painful, for many of the residents had been in Plymouth during the Blitz and all had witnessed the effects.

"That music – we were dancing to the same tunes on the Hoe," said Mrs Bennett, "and one night the pier and all its beautiful glass and metalwork was there; next evening, we were dancing among the rubble and the pier was a burnt-out twisted shell."

Mrs Tremayne spoke. "It wasn't just what Gerry's bombs destroyed. It was the fear and people and little children screaming. And you weren't safe even in the shelters, were you? Remember when the shelter at Portland Square was hit? They didn't bury them, you know. They just covered over the ruins of the shelter."

Mrs Austin surprised Gemma with the clarity and detail of her memories. "It wasn't even just all the dead and injured. It was night after night the sirens, the droning of the German bombers, the ack-ack fire, the thud and roar of the explosives; the fires burning all night in the city, the smell of brick dust and cordite in the morning; and we didn't know if it would ever end."

"People looking for their relatives…"

"People looking for their homes…"

George said, "After I was wounded, they brought me back to Plymouth. So many bodies. At the height of the Blitz, those dustcarts going round picking up bodies. They'd put a shroud over them but sometimes you could recognize them." His voice was scarcely audible. "Sometimes you'd see children's shoes and feet sticking out."

"That was the lowest point for me," said Mrs Bennett, "when they had to start digging mass graves."

Beatrice spoke. "That's where they put my Daniel – in a mass grave up at Efford."

There was a silence – of sympathy, but surprise, too, because most of the residents had never heard Beatrice talk. Gemma, except for her laments on the beach, could only ever remember her making that comment about it being sad when people quarrel when Matron sacked Nurse Thompson.

Then Mrs Tremayne said, "You know, I think people born after the war, who didn't have to live through it, don't know what horror, true horror, is." People nodded in agreement.

And Gemma was surprised again by Mrs Austin, who said, "They say, 'Forgive and forget.' You can forgive, because life moves on and it becomes silly to keep hating. Forget – they say, 'It's fifty years ago.' But it isn't – it's like it was yesterday; and you don't forget yesterday."

There was another silence. Then Mr Mitchell spoke. With his indistinct speech they had to strain to hear. "I don't want to hear no bull about the wartime spirit. We did what we did because we had no choice. We reckoned that you had to muck in together or get conquered and starve – those they hadn't killed first. Those were our choices. But one memory that stays with me was after they'd bombed St Andrew's – those terrible air-raids of March 1941. When we heard that they'd got our church, we went down to see for ourselves. Like you were saying –" he looked at Mrs Austin "– you had to get through the rubble and all the dust and dirt in the air; and the smell of burning from the incendiaries and the buildings with their fronts out... Anyway we got there and there was a well-dressed woman there with a sign saying 'Resurgam' – that's 'I shall rise again'," he explained to Gemma. "And she wanted to put this sign on the door frame of the church – the door itself had been blown in – but she'd only got this puny little hammer and that wasn't going to make any effect on the old lintel, so this squaddie in his army greatcoat picked up a large stone – a bit of the old church – from among all the rubble; and he takes the sign and the nail from her in one hand and he takes this dirty great piece of stone in the other and smashes the nail through the sign into the lintel."

He stopped, exhausted. Little more was said after that. People wandered away. Mrs Bennett was one of the last. As she went, she grasped both of Gemma's hands together and said to her, "You know, we saw lots of bad things in our time. But we mustn't let that make us give up – we must protect the good."

The Corporal and George stayed on to help Gemma wash and tidy up. The light was fading. The Corporal looked out of the windows at the working lights of the fishing boats pulling in their nets, the powerful pulse of the Eddystone light and the red blink of Fishertown pierhead light. "It was on a day like this in 1945," he said quietly, "that I came back on the troopship to Southampton. That's where they discharged me. They gave me a demob suit and ten pounds and a railway ticket home. So I got off at Millbay but the city I'd left wasn't there anymore. The skyline was all wrong; the roads didn't go anywhere. And, when eventually I got home, my wife was someone I hadn't seen for five years; she just wasn't the same woman I'd married; and the baby I'd left behind was now six years old –" his voice dropped "– and he didn't recognize me. He asked his mum 'Who's this man?' and when she said, 'It's your dad, of course,' I could see he didn't believe her.

"You couldn't talk to the civilians about your war. They'd had their own war and that had been bad enough and they didn't want to talk about it any more. They wanted to forget it. So I'd go drinking with my old schoolmates – those that were still alive – and we'd all get plastered and say how it had been a good war; and all the time I'd be thinking, What did I fight for? What did I kill for? and it didn't make sense; and I'd have these bad dreams and relive my chums being blown up in front of me and having to find the bits so that we had something to put in their graves."

"Yes," said George, "I remember that – putting bits of your mates into body bags. Half the time you didn't have a clue whose arm or leg was whose."

"Anyway, like you, George," the Corporal went on, "I got work. There was work to be had rebuilding the city and I was always good with my hands. But at home I was a little dictator, couldn't help myself – losing my rag at the slightest thing; if anything didn't go just right, the way I wanted it done, yelling and shouting and sometimes hitting her and him…" He paused. "The boy left home as soon as he could. Just walked out one day when he was eighteen. The wife, she put up with me. When she got ill, I tried to say sorry, and she said she knew I'd never really meant it." He started to cry. "Of course I hadn't meant it but I couldn't stop myself. It was like I was hollow inside but trying to pretend I was still real. And then she got ill." He had buried his face in his hands and was sobbing. Gemma wanted to go and comfort him but she hung back. George went over and put his arm round him. The Corporal went on sobbing and then, between sobs, he whispered, "And then the ambulance took her to hospital... By the time I got there... So I never could say, never really did say sorry." He sat silent, his head in his hands, rocking slightly.

George spoke. "Lots of ex-servicemen were like that," he said. "The war did that to us; it never really ended. We kept on being at war in our heads, waiting for the whistle of the next bullet, the one with our name on it. Don't blame yourself. Blame the war."

The Corporal looked at him. "Do you mean that?"

"Of course I do."

"You really mean that?" The Corporal still didn't seem to believe him.

George looked at him steadily. "I said I do."

The Corporal turned away; and stared dully at the lights flickering out at sea. "So it's over, the war – it's really over?"

George patted him on the back. The Corporal wiped his eyes and then said, "Well, if it's over, it's pretty daft calling me Corporal, isn't it? They baptized me Terence, but everyone called me Terry."

"Terry," said George. "That's a nice name. Had a dog once called Terry."

After George and Terry had said goodnight and left her, Gemma felt confused. The wild exuberance of the dance had now been darkened by the residents' so-vivid memories of the war and its aftermath. And yet the spontaneity and the enjoyment of the dance had seemed so genuine.

Her shift had now finished, so she changed and went out to *Periwinkle*. She undid the lines and launched her into the dusk-rimmed sea, and let the boat float gently in the evening breeze.

After a while, she felt calmer. She brought *Periwinkle* ashore and pulled her up the beach, near to where the bandstand stood, waiting to be dismantled. It was a soft, warm night so she decided to sleep outside. She went into the Beacon and said hello and a few words to Mrs Tremayne who was sitting in the lounge. Then she got her sleeping bag and went out. She positioned *Periwinkle* to act as a windshield, for she had learnt that even a light breeze was cold at dawn and woke you shivering. Then she rolled out the groundsheet and the sleeping bag.

It only seemed a few minutes later that she was woken by someone moving around and whispering her name. There was no light to see by. "Who is it? What do you want?" she called out.

"It's me, Mrs Tremayne. Here's the key to my room – please get my cello."

Gemma slipped wearily out of her sleeping bag. She could now see the outline of Mrs Tremayne. She helped her to a chair on the bandstand and got her safely seated. She went inside, found Mrs Tremayne's cello case and brought it outside. She opened the case. Mrs Tremayne took the cello and the bow. She tuned it. "Elgar," she said and then began to play. The music poured out and rolled into the still air. It was deep, plaintive music that was infinitely sad and lonely. As Mrs Tremayne played, the first rays of light broke across the blackness of the night sky to the east and then the red lip of the sun rose slowly over Rame.

Chapter Eleven

Appointment in Truro

On Lantern Beach there were no trees dropping their brown and golden leaves to mark the arrival of autumn; instead, the little black-headed terns no longer fluttered along the tideline and, after each rainy day, the earth did not warm up quite as much as before, as if the sun, now lower in the sky, had lost its power to heal. Gemma still sailed when she could, and she usually went with Tom. They would explore some of the smaller bays and hollows, and Tom would show her where he had gone crabbing, and which rocks the crabs hid under. And they'd go ashore and he'd talk about the fishing – how, when barely in his teens, he'd started working on his father's boat; of catches so big you could hardly pull the nets in; how, if you weren't careful fishing inshore, you could get caught as the tide went out; and if you grounded on rock, the waves would pound the keel so bad few boats ever got off; almost all were wrecks by the morning.

In September, an appointment at the hospital arrived for Mrs Bennett. "Good to see the consultant's back from his holiday," said Rose. "It'll be to tell you the results of all those tests you did." Mrs Bennett asked Gemma if she would come with her. So, on the day of the appointment, they left early to make the long journey. It involved a bus, a small local train from Fishertown to the main line station and then another train and another bus to the hospital.

Eventually they were called into the doctor's office. He was wearing a dark suit. He had Mrs Bennett's X-rays and test results on the desk in front of him. He placed the X-rays against a lit screen and studied them for a minute in silence. He turned and sat down again. "Mrs Bennett? You're here for your results. Well, I'm sorry to have to tell you that they show the cancer is still active." Gemma felt Mrs Bennett reach for her hand and and squeeze it. "*But* we should be able to slow it down – or with a bit of luck even stop it – if you have some surgery as soon as possible, and then a course of treatment for a few months after that." He paused enquiringly.

Mrs Bennett looked at the X-rays of her body lit up on the screen and then at him. "That's very kind, but no, thank you."

The doctor tried to persuade her, but Mrs Bennett was sure – no treatment. The doctor shrugged, told her he would write to her GP and his nurse showed them out.

Gemma was surprised at Mrs Bennett's decision but didn't think it was her place to say so. Death, or a longer life. That had to be Mrs Bennett's choice. When eventually they had got onto the local train down to Fishertown, Mrs Bennett explained. "I saw my husband have the treatment, but I wasn't going to tell the doctor that – none of his business. I cared for him for those last three years. I saw him change from a strong, healthy man to an old, shrunken skeleton. All the treatment did was to prolong his suffering. When your time comes… I'm happy now. The Beacon's been good to me. It is good to me. I don't want to cling onto life by my fingernails…"

Gemma nodded, and said nothing, and watched the river and the woods roll past outside the window.

Chapter Twelve

Ocean Bay

The autumn equinox – that time in September when night becomes as long as day and often there are great gales – had passed. It was time to start thinking about getting *Periwinkle* out of the water. Gemma had found a boatyard in Fishertown where she could store her safely over the winter. "I think I'll do one more trip before I take her out," she said to Tom one day. He nodded. "I was thinking of Ocean Bay." Ocean Bay was a few miles west of Fishertown.

"You be careful of Ocean Bay," said Tom. "It's easy enough to get into but if the wind's at all onshore, it can be the very devil to get out of. So just you be careful." Gemma promised she would.

She had a day off during the week, packed some sandwiches and a spare set of clothing and was soon heading west. The brisk southerly wind allowed her to sail quickly down the coast.

Ocean Bay came in view. It was formed by a large circular beach backed by very steep cliffs. Gemma turned *Periwinkle* inshore and the boat, its sails filled, screamed towards the beach. Soon she was in the breakers, the white water hissing along the top of the collapsing waves. Just before she hit the beach, Gemma swung *Periwinkle* around into the wind and leapt out. *Periwinkle's* sails juddered and banged as she pulled the boat backwards up the sand.

She sat down cross-legged on some dry sand behind a rock, to get some shelter from the wind. She had been at the Beacon eight months now. Sometimes she wondered if she should do something different, if she should move on. Mrs O'Halloran was encouraging her to study and to think about going to college, but because she hadn't done well at school, she was a bit afraid of risking herself with books and essays. Besides, she was enjoying her work, learning from what the residents had taught her – that people could still use their skills and could pass them on. Tom had taught her so much. Even if they had difficulties, people could still function with help, like Mrs Austin with Kathy. And Mrs Austin had times when she startled Gemma with her understanding, like the night after the concert. She was learning how important communication was to keeping you alive and involved, as was Mr Mitchell, despite the effort it was for him to talk and be heard. Mrs Bennett had taught her that you could prepare yourself for dying, so that you met death with dignity and in peace.

And George – she had heard long, uncontrollable bouts of coughing coming from his room. She suspected that he was feeling increasingly fragile, and that he wanted to make his peace with the world. She could see more clearly now how the parts of people's lives fitted together and made sense of who they were, what they believed and what they did now – as Beatrice's grief and her wanting to be alone on the beach went together; but even when you were old, you could still shape or reshape your destiny, as Martha Tremayne and Terry were doing.

And she, too, could choose who she was and what she would be. Of course she shouldn't leave while the residents were teaching her so much. She needn't worry about when the right time would be to leave – it wasn't something that she could judge by using other people's values. No-one could tell her, impose their time on her. Besides, it was wrong to think of time as something that you must never waste. It wasn't like water in the desert. She would know when it was time to move on. And maybe when it was time – if she and Adam were still together – she'd be ready to take up his offer and ride pillion to London and whatever the city held for her.

Right now she was starving. She got the sandwiches she'd made earlier out from the locker beneath *Periwinkle*'s mast and sat on the sand munching them. They tasted very good as she wolfed them down.

The sun was lower in the sky and the wind definitely felt stronger. She had to leave very soon if she was to get back to Lantern Beach before nightfall. There was no-one else on the beach. Out to sea, all she could see and hear were the white, breaking, rolling waves. She turned and looked behind her. The cliff-face was practically sheer. There must surely be a path down to the beach but she couldn't see one – just green and purple gorse and the odd stunted tree as the cliff towered high above her. Birds floated in the thermals at the cliff edge – seagulls to judge by their mewing calls, but she couldn't tell as they were little larger than black dots.

She turned back towards the sea, where the breakers rolled in, large, relentless and close together. The noise as they crashed and collapsed was deafening.

She had to get *Periwinkle* through them. She remembered Tom's advice with chagrin – "Beware an onshore wind" – and here she was with the wind blowing her hair backwards.

She had to try. Even if she could find the path up the cliffs, she had brought no money with her, so it would be a long walk in the dark back to Fishertown, and she couldn't leave *Periwinkle* on this strange beach. At high tide, she would probably be smashed against the cliffs.

She brought *Periwinkle* down to the water's edge, and hoisted the mainsail. Then she tentatively pushed the boat into the water. She heard the hissing of a large wave coming towards her. It broke and sizzled around her, picked *Periwinkle* up, threw her sideways, tore Gemma's feet away from the bottom and, with effortless scorn, threw them both back on the shore whilst it died in a carpet of foam higher up the beach.

Gemma got back on her feet. *Periwinkle* – thank God – was undamaged, although she was on her side, a mass of sodden sails and ropes. She took the mast and pulled the boat upright. Like a dog shaking itself, the water drained away from it.

She was soaked and shaken. Wearing her buoyancy aid, she shouldn't drown, but if she got caught in the ropes, knocked unconscious by the mast, or if she was thrown out of the boat in the deeper water and there were undercurrents, then she could suffocate or drown. How stupid, stupid, stupid she had been! How many times had Tom said to her, "Before you sail, go down to the sea. Look at it – and the sky. Listen to it – and the wind. Give it time to talk to you and you'll know what it'll be like out there." Instead she'd just pulled *Periwinkle* down to the water and taken off. If only she'd listened to his advice, listened to his experience.

She knew she only had the strength in her for one last attempt to get away from the beach. She took off her soaked clothes and wrung out the water. They chilled her as she put them back on. She walked up the beach, away from the power of the waves to give herself time to work out the best strategy. She wondered what Adam would do, and remembered how he had once described getting off a beach in *Periwinkle* by diving aboard at the very last minute.

Again, she pulled *Periwinkle* down to the water line. She positioned herself amidships and this time, holding her boat, ran much faster into the sea and, as the first breaker reared up above her, held on and kept moving out. The breaker roared and broke across *Periwinkle* and filled Gemma's mouth with salt water and blinded her eyes into a grey, stinging blur; but Gemma knew she had to hold the boat facing out to the sea, fighting with all her might against the breaking wave's attempt to throw *Periwinkle* sidewards and backwards. The wave frothed and then was past her.

The next wave was starting to enlarge. It was swelling; the blue of its top became the grey of its belly. It was starting to rear up. She had only a few seconds to get in and get control of the boat. Now! She threw herself into the boat and slithered across the bottom, ignoring the pain of the contact. For a fleeting second, a phrase that she had heard up at St Keverne's flashed through her mind: "The Lord giveth and the Lord taketh away." She threw herself onto the far side of the dinghy, turned, grabbed the tiller with one hand and found the wet mainsheet with the other. Then she angled the boat up to the wind. The wave grew nearer still. It reared up before her. Just before it reached the boat, she threw *Periwinkle* head to wind. The water roared and powered over the boat, which climbed up, up into the air – Gemma held onto the boom to stop herself falling backwards into the mad, foaming surf – and then *Periwinkle* was falling and smashed down on the back of the wave. The wave rushed onwards, breaking as it went. Gemma eased off the wind, and gained a few more metres from the shore. The next breaker had a bit more depth of water beneath it so was less fierce as Gemma again headed into it at the last moment. Once more, water poured along the boat and over her, but with a little less venom.

In another few minutes, she was through the breakers. White horses rode the wave tops but in an orderly fashion. She was alive to tell the tale, but she was too cold and wet to feel exultant. She just recognized that she was now safe and would live – and live to admit ruefully to Tom that his advice had been all too accurate.

Soon she was able to turn the boat sidewards to the wind and start heading swiftly back to Lantern Beach. Holding the tiller with one hand, she reached forward into the locker beneath the mast for the bag of dry clothes and a towel. During the next few minutes she wriggled out of her damp clothes, dried her goose-pimpled flesh and put the dry ones on. She even found a piece of chocolate to eat, so was feeling much calmer as she approached Lantern Bay. It was now early evening and the wind had dropped to little more than a breeze as she brought *Periwinkle* ashore.

Tom had been waiting and watching out for her. He came down to the waves to help her drag *Periwinkle* up the beach. "I was worried for you and *Periwinkle*, Maid Gemma," he said. Gemma knew she didn't have to tell

Tom what she'd been through. She knew he already knew. She dropped the rope she had been using to drag *Periwinkle* to safety, put her arms around Tom and gave him a big kiss on the cheek and then stayed there silently, glad to be alive, hugging him and being hugged in return.

Chapter Thirteen

Storm

The days continued to draw in.

Despite the days getting shorter and colder, Tom and Beatrice still patrolled their parts of the beach. The staff made sure they were warm and asked them to come in if it got too cold.

Gemma had intended to sail *Periwinkle* home on the first fine day that she had free. But now the sky had been grey for days with small scudding black clouds running east underneath it. The Eddystone had long been lost in a blanket of dirty white mist. The sun shone an unhealthy yellow and there was a bright white ring around it. The sea was sullen. Its blue had turned to a grey soup. Further out in the bay there was a big swell. Experienced heads in the Lookout that evening warned of bad weather.

Gemma took all the gear that might blow away or be damaged off the boat and put it, for safety, in one of the home's sheds; she pulled *Periwinkle* to the top of the beach, and then secured her with strong ropes.

After supper, the wind started to rise. It started whining around the Beacon trying to find a way in – any way in – against the door, through the windows or down the ventilators. The sound made the residents restless. They didn't want to go to bed and those that did soon gave up trying to sleep and got up again. But anxious as they were, tiredness came on them and eventually all had settled down to a restless slumber.

Gemma was sleeping in that night. Barbara was on duty. Gemma, too, had difficulty getting off to sleep. She got up and made herself some cocoa, and sat at a table with Mr Mitchell and Mrs Austin. Barbara joined them. Making talk to drown out the howling and screaming of the wind from their minds, Mr Mitchell asked her why she had come to the Beacon from up-country.

Barbara replied, "I've been in this kind of work for some years. I was working in a local authority home and they kept telling us that all these changes were improvements, but we at the sharp end knew things were actually getting worse and worse. I didn't have any family commitments – my children had grown up and moved out. In the end, I had to get out to keep my self-respect, and to have some job satisfaction. So I started looking around. My parents used to bring us children – my brother and I – down to Fishertown for holidays, so I knew this neck of the woods, and when this job came up, I thought, OK – let's give it a go."

They finished their cocoa. Gemma went back to bed and tried to get to sleep again, but the wind seemed to be getting stronger. The whistling had stopped. Now there was a moaning, then a pause, and then another moan. And then the rain came. It hit her window like pistol shots. It was impossible to sleep. All she could do was doze.

Some time later, someone was shaking her. It was Barbara.

"Tom's not in his bed. I've looked all round. I can't find him."

Gemma dressed as quickly as possible. She went round the whole building. The night lights were on. She could see by their bluish illumination. There was no sign of Tom. She was coming back through the central area when there was a bang as the main door to the building crashed open. Gemma realized it would not have done that if it was locked.

Tom must have unlocked it when he'd gone out.

She seized a torch from the wall – she had to find Tom. She found the nearest coat, threw it on and went through the open door. The wind nearly drove her back inside. The rain stung her face and her eyes so hard it was painful to keep them open. She was soaked in seconds.

Beach and sea were one. There was no separation. The waves were tumbling over each other and rushing up the beach. They were foaming and spurting onwards till they reached the wall on the side of the road, reared up and then frothed backwards. All the time there was the sound of the sea roaring and panting. Gemma was very scared, all too aware of the power of the sea to tear her away from the land and throw her into a whirlpool of death.

The air was full of spume and spray. The bullets of rain made Gemma want to cough and gasp. The only way she could make any progress along the beach was with her back to the wind.

The wind was not just very powerful, making walking difficult and making Gemma crouch as she moved; its howling was almost human. The howls were howls of rage and anger – this was a wind seeking vengeance.

And still no Tom.

The force of the wind seemed to hold her as if refusing to let her move another yard. Gemma walked along the top of the beach, casting the torch beam around to see if he was perhaps somewhere in the surf. Then she tripped.

She realized that she had tripped over the ropes securing Periwinkle.

She shone her torch. *Periwinkle* was covered by sand, which to a small extent was protecting the boat.

Then she saw something sticking out from under *Periwinkle*. A hand. It had to be Tom's. She tried to lift

Periwinkle up. The wind smashed it down again. But in that second she saw Tom lying there.

She realized it was pointless trying to lift and hold the dinghy up. The best she could achieve was to tip it over and away from Tom. She put both hands underneath *Periwinkle*, waited for a slight lull in the wind and then gave a great heave to upturn *Periwinkle* and release Tom. The dinghy resisted for the first few inches but, as she came up, the wind turned from persecutor to helper and flipped her over.

Tom was lying very still. Was he breathing? Gemma had been taught first aid when she started at the Beacon but, in these conditions, with all the noise and foam in the air, it was impossible to tell. She had to get Tom inside, into the warm. But he was unable to help her. She picked him up under his shoulders and slowly dragged his wiry frame along the beach. Thank God he wasn't any heavier, but it was very difficult for Gemma as she was now facing into the gale and the air was still full of driving rain that attacked her face, her eyes and her mouth, and made it hard for her to breathe.

Slowly, she pulled him a yard or two at a time and then had to rest. Gradually, she came into the lights of the Beacon. Once she'd got him inside the surrounding wall, there was a bit of shelter; and then Barbara, who'd been waiting and watching by a window, came out to help them through the front door. "God, you've been brave," she said, but Gemma was past acknowledging praise. Once indoors, Barbara bent down and checked Tom's breathing and pulse. "He'll live," she said.

They took off his wet clothes, put him in a warm bath and gave him warm tea. Gradually his colour returned. They dried him, got him in his pyjamas and into bed.

Gemma was exhausted as she had never been before. Every muscle ached. The simplest thought took an age. But she had to make sure Tom was all right before she could let herself sleep, so she told Barbara she'd sit with him for a bit.

Tom settled down and then opened his eyes. "I'm sorry, Maid Gemma; I had to check she was all right."

Soon, he was asleep; his breathing was soft and regular. Gemma was too tired to rise, and it was Barbara who gently helped her to her bed and tucked her in.

Chapter Fourteen

Light Fading

Mrs Bennett was getting weaker. She had trouble walking now and was falling more often. She was also getting more confused. She'd say she was back in Plymouth, or talk to Gemma at one time as if she was her daughter, and at another time, as if she was talking to her mother. It was clear to everyone, including herself, that the cancer had spread.

She spent more and more time in her room. There were letters that she wanted to write. Each one, though not more than a few lines, took many hours of difficult concentration. Often she was grateful for Gemma's help in finishing them.

One afternoon, she went to bed for a nap. On waking and taking an afternoon cup of tea, she asked Gemma if she would take her to the Lookout that evening and if the other residents could be there. So Gemma and Rose helped her to bath. Then Mrs Bennett chose the dress she wanted to wear and the make-up and the jewellery to match.

When she was finished, she looked at herself in the mirror, and then carefully dabbed her favourite perfume behind her ears and on her wrists. "I'm ready," she said.

They put her in a wheelchair, for she was now too weak to walk any distance, and took her to the lift.

The Lookout was full of sunlight. Word had been spread of Mrs Bennett's wish and all the residents were there. Mrs Bennett said clearly, but weakly, that she wanted to buy everyone a drink. There were protestations but these were ignored.

Gemma served the drinks. When everyone had got one, there was a hush as they waited for Mrs Bennett to offer a toast. She raised her glass; "To the future."

"To the future," they replied. Uneasy at the thought that they were toasting the future with a dying woman, nevertheless each, in turn, came over and clinked a glass with hers. Mrs Austin was the last. She looked rather confused and bewildered as she came near. She touched Mrs Bennett on the arm and then began weeping. Mrs Bennett reached out from her wheelchair towards her and they embraced.

The sun was still high above the horizon as Gemma took Mrs Bennett back to her room. "That was good," she said, "but I am very tired."

She was now needing strong painkillers. The doctor tried to prescribe medicine that took away the pain without dulling her ability to think or to feel. Nurse

Barratt, who had replaced Nurse Thompson, had worked in a hospice, a unit whose purpose was to help people die with dignity and without unnecessary pain. She stayed on for many extra hours to make sure that the drugs were working. She also arranged for Mrs Bennett to have regular massages and used aroma-therapy to provide a soothing atmosphere to the room. Gemma found her expertise reassuring, because it gave a bit of control to Mrs Bennett in her journey towards death.

There came the day when Mrs Bennett no longer left her bed, except to be helped to the toilet. "It won't be long now," she said to Gemma. "I'll be glad."

Rose and Gemma were quietly talking in the lounge area when Martha Tremayne came up to them. "I don't know if it's the right thing but I was wondering – do you think she'd like some music?"

Rose answered, "Why don't we try and see?"

Gemma got Mrs Tremayne's cello and carried it to Mrs Bennett's room. Then she got her a chair. Mrs Tremayne started playing quietly "Abide with Me", an old Methodist chapel hymn. Mrs Bennett stirred and Mrs Tremayne stopped playing. Mrs Bennett leant towards Gemma who was sitting by her side. "Tell her to go on," she said, weakly but clearly.

It became evident that Mrs Tremayne remembered all the tunes she'd played to her charges in the school those many years ago. Hymns, folk songs, nursery rhymes, simple piano pieces, she played them all for Mrs

Bennett. And because Mrs Bennett found them soothing and comforting, Mrs Tremayne would play for her for a while every morning and afternoon; and when she played, somehow it stopped being sad in that room of dying, and became almost serene and joyous.

Gemma spent nearly all her time helping Mrs Bennett, but there was often little to do because Mrs Bennett spent much of her time asleep.

Rose helped Gemma keep the pillows plumped up and the scented candles, which Mrs Bennett liked, burning; and helped with washing and turning her over every few hours to prevent her skin getting sore.

Mrs Bennett started to lose her appetite, but what worried Rose more was her difficulty swallowing water. "You take a long time starving to death; lack of fluids is what kills you," she told Gemma.

Still Mrs Bennett continued to take little food or fluid. She had now lost so much weight that Gemma could see her ribs and when she took her hand, she could feel the bones in her wrist. But her stomach was hard and swollen from the growth of the cancer. Her skin was tinted yellow, telling Nurse Barratt that her liver was no longer functioning properly. "Are you sure you want to go on with this, Gemma?" she asked one day.

Gemma did want to go on. The silences got longer. She heard Mrs Bennett apologize one night for being such a nuisance – heard her say "Thank you" in the middle of another long night.

It was like her Nan all over again, but this time Gemma knew she was able to help Mrs Bennett die in comfort and dignity. In those long silences, she would think of visits to her Nan and feel sad, helpless and angry that her Nan had had to die in such squalor.

Mrs Tremayne faithfully came to play for Mrs Bennett each day, but there came a day when the music had lost its power to arouse her or to soothe her and give her pleasure.

She was also on yet more painkillers after some disturbed nights and the doctor was asked to visit again. As he left, he warned Rose that it was quite likely that Mrs Bennett might not live for more than another forty-eight hours.

Gemma was determined to be with Mrs Bennett to the end. She sat by her bedside and held her hand. She mopped her brow with a wet flannel and kept her lips moist.

Towards the end, the only time Gemma left the room was when residents came in to say their goodbyes.

Day turned into night. Mrs Bennett slept and stirred. Gemma watched her, watched over her and felt herself getting more and more tired. She fought off sleep but her eyelids grew heavy and sleep came.

Someone was gently shaking her shoulder. "It's over, Gemma. It's all over and it was peaceful." It was Rose.

Gemma was angry. "I should have been there. You should have kept me awake. It was so wrong of me to fall asleep."

"No, it was only when you had fallen asleep that she could go. Mrs Bennett knew how much you wanted her to live, so she couldn't let you down by dying whilst you were awake."

It took a long time for Gemma to understand that and to forgive herself.

Chapter Fifteen

Two White Horses

Mrs Bennett lay in her room for twenty-four hours so that all could visit her and pay their last respects.

One of the customs of the Beacon was that the residents helped arrange a funeral. If relatives were sorting things out, then the residents would try and offer them comfort and support. In Mrs Bennett's case, her daughter was unable to get over from Australia, so the residents had to make the arrangements. Mrs O'Halloran told them that Mrs Bennett had asked that she be buried near the Beacon, where she had felt at home and with friends, and the vicar of St Keverne was agreeable. She had left enough money for a proper funeral; Mrs O'Halloran also told them that no-one new would be admitted till they felt ready to welcome them.

When the residents had all paid their respects, they got together to discuss the funeral arrangements.

"A celebration of life, not a death," said Mrs Tremayne.

"She needs a funeral procession even if we have to hire a Boy Scout troop to push us there," said George.

"The service in the Authorized Version and not modern slang," added Mr Mitchell.

Tom wanted the service outside. "Being cooped up inside a church gives me the willies."

"And a vicar who knows who he's talking about," said Terry, with feeling. "I had to listen to a vicar talking about the wife of an old mate of mine once. 'Gentle, kindly soul,' he said. Well, the woman had the most vicious tongue I've ever heard…"

So gradually they worked out the details, asked the local vicar to come in and agree on the service and told him all they knew about Mrs Bennett and what she meant to them.

They asked Gemma to go up to St Winnow, where Mrs Bennett had come from, and put a notice in the village shop inviting her friends to come to the funeral. So the next day, Gemma cycled over. It was quite a long ride and she was glad when she was finally cycling down the hill into the village. The shopkeeper remembered Mrs Bennett well. He was happy to put a notice up and to pass the word around. He was sure if they could sort out transport, some of her old friends would want to attend her funeral. After her mission had been accomplished, Gemma walked down through the village churchyard that was at the water's edge and stood by the lazily flowing river, remembering Mrs Bennett and letting the sunlight warm her body after its long vigil. The river widened into a small lake by the village, and in its centre a man in a rowing boat was fishing. Behind her, cows in a barn were mooing. She picked a yellow flower from the bank, threw it in the water, and watched it slowly drift downstream. She felt at peace.

Mrs Bennett had spent her childhood here, so when she was a little child all those years ago, she would have stood on this spot by the river. Gemma could almost see this child, in a Victorian smock, beside her now, looking with big eyes across the water. She smiled, shook the thought from her head and walked back through the graveyard crosses to her bike.

As the residents wanted the service to be out of doors if at all possible, it was lucky that the day of the funeral turned out fine. The mourners assembled in a car park a couple of hundred yards from the church. Gemma was pleased to see a minivan of mourners arrive from St Winnow. Terry had rung the local school, and a number of schoolchildren had volunteered to help at the funeral.

From down the hill came the sound of a marching band. "George's idea," whispered Terry to Gemma.

"My daughter took me to Fishertown last Sunday lunchtime for a drink," George told her. "There was this jazz band playing in the pub and I asked them if they thought they could do a funeral."

The band came towards the mourners. Behind the band was a cart covered in a white cloth, on which was the coffin, also draped in white. On top of the coffin were lilies. The cart was being pulled by two beautiful white horses.

The band moved off at a slow pace down the street playing a dirge, followed by the horses pulling Mrs Bennett's coffin, then the mourners, some of whom needed a bit of help from the schoolchildren. As they got to the cemetery by the church, the gates were swung open, and the horses and coffin went through, disturbing the church cat asleep in the cemetery hedge. They stopped at the grave, freshly dug with brown earth piled up on its sides. There the mourners were greeted by the vicar.

"At your request this service is being held outside," he said, and then he talked for a few minutes about Mrs Bennett and how her life was now complete because death did not so much end life as complete it. Death was part of life and gave it meaning.

Then the vicar began the service and the great, resonant verses of the Authorized Version rolled out across the graveyard under the yews – "Oh death where is thy sting? Oh grave where is thy victory?" – until the vicar recited, "Earth to earth, ashes to ashes, dust to dust," and the coffin was lowered into the grave, still with its white cloth, and its lilies. A single bell tolled in the tower of the church.

The congregation edged forward and each member threw a handful of earth into the grave. Gemma watched each one as they paid their last respects. So far she had felt composed, but now, at this final parting, tears started running down her face. She hadn't wanted them to, but there was nothing she could do to stop them. Embarrassed, she took out her handkerchief and covered her eyes, and then she knew that she too had to acknowledge that Mrs Bennett really was dead and she would never see or talk to her again. Pushing the handkerchief into her pocket, she stepped forward, took the trowel with a hand that trembled and threw earth onto the solid wooden lid of Mrs Bennett's coffin.

When all were done, there was a silence as the congregation remembered not only Mrs Bennett but also all those who mattered to them who had died before her.

With a little cough, the vicar brought them back to the present, telling them he had an announcement to make.

Apparently, before she became seriously ill, Mrs Bennett had made a request to Mrs O'Halloran that, after the funeral, there should be a luncheon. No expense should be spared and if people wanted to get a bit jolly, that was fine by her, and that included the vicar.

At this, there was much laughter, which helped reduce the tension that comes with a funeral. And the vicar made one last request. "I know Mrs Bennett would have wanted your lives to go on. She has finished hers but you must go about your daily business. I would like us to give strength to each other. Can I ask that you all greet each other – a hug or handshake and a few words, perhaps 'Go in peace', so we share and bear our sorrow between us?"

The congregation found that to be a strange request and the first few handshakes and arms on shoulders were stiff, especially as the vicar had joined them, but gradually they relaxed and could see the purpose in what they were doing: that they could and should trust each other in sharing the sad present and an unknown future.

When all were done, the musicians sprang to life and, with a lively tune, led the mourners into the adjoining field. And there was Steve and the schoolchildren. They had quietly been putting out trestle tables during the service, which they had been able to hear and follow over the hedge. The tables were loaded with every kind of delicacy the residents liked – pasties, hams, meats – laid out on fine linen tablecloths, and such a myriad variety of alcoholic and non-alcoholic drinks as to shame an off-licence. "Now this," said Terry to George, as they helped themselves to a plateful and a glass, "is what I call a spread."

And the horses brought the cart into the field and started munching on its rich green grass, and the band members climbed onto the cart and began to play the jazz music they usually played on Sundays in the pub.

In this way was the life of Mrs Bennett celebrated.

Chapter Sixteen

The View from the Cliff

After the funeral, Gemma had to sort out *Periwinkle*. The storm had caused some damage to her planking and the rigging but, with Tom's help and advice, they were able to mend it; and as soon as it was fixed, she sailed *Periwinkle* back to Fishertown and took her out of the water for the winter. That way, she could be sure that Tom was not going to put himself at risk looking after her.

Tom himself had recovered but he was definitely weaker. He still spent most of his time outside but he was slower and less safe on his feet.

One night during this time, Gemma was on duty. A couple of the residents had got up in the night and a cup of cocoa seemed a good idea – except that there wasn't any in the cupboard. So she got the key and went to the stores. As she came into the central area she could see that someone was sitting in the office in the dark. Gemma quietly turned the light on.

It was the Matron and she was staring straight ahead.

"Are you all right, Mrs O'Halloran?"

Mrs O'Halloran turned. "Yes – well…" Her voice trembled slightly. "I mean…" She seemed lost in her own thoughts. "Did I ever tell you I worked in a mission school in Africa?" Gemma shook her head. "We were doing good work; you could see the villagers' health was getting better every year and the children were doing really well at their lessons. And we had one orphan child, so we had him live with us and he helped out – Afinicki was his name. I got fond of him. Then the civil war came. And one day soldiers surrounded the village and before we had time to hide Afinicki, they had found him. Their leader came up to me and he said they were taking him away to give him a proper political upbringing and that he'd come back when there was peace. I knew that wasn't at all what he meant, but he was swinging an automatic rifle in case I got difficult. So I just had to watch as they took him away…" Her voice broke. "I'm sorry," she said. "It's not your fault. It's really nothing that you've done. It's man's inhumanity to man that I can never get used to." Then she got up and quickly left the room.

The incident puzzled and bothered Gemma – it was so unlike Mrs O'Halloran – but this puzzlement was swept away by the arrival of her eighteenth birthday.

On the day of her birthday, after the daily meeting, a cake made by the residents and a large card were suddenly produced and everyone sang "Happy birthday, dear Gemma." And when the singing ended, Tom, with an embarrassed grin, pushed a paper bag into her hand. "This is from all of us."

Gemma took the bag. In it was a box created from wood made white by the sea. On its top Tom had burnt in the letters GEMMA. She stared at it. "It's beautiful. It must have taken you hours to make."

"It did," said George. "Would you like to open it?" Gemma opened the box and inside was a silver bracelet with the greenest stones.

"It's just like you, Gemma," Beatrice said. "Very precious."

She wasn't working the next day. When she got home, to her surprise she found her mother in her slip in front of her dressing table mirror, getting ready to go out. "If I can't celebrate my only daughter's eighteenth…" she said, as she carefully applied her eyeshadow. So Gemma felt she too had to dress in her finest. "Mum, you look really glam," Gemma said as they walked arm in arm to a nearby pub.

Roy, the landlord, who had known them for years, personally ushered them to a table in the candle-lit restaurant room. Gemma couldn't remember a time when she and her mum had gone out to eat in style like this and felt a bit proud. She almost felt shy, worrying about whether she would find enough to say to her mother all evening.

But it wasn't a problem. She took the present and two cards that she had got for her birthday out of her handbag and showed them to her mother. One was from the residents and the other from Mrs O'Halloran, in which she had written, "I'm so glad I was given the chance to spot your talent that day in the café. Thank you for bringing life and light into the Beacon." Her mum was most impressed and wanted to hear all about what was happening at the Beacon and then, over a glass of wine, she started to tell Gemma stories of when she was younger. And, inevitably, her dad got mentioned.

For the first time, Gemma felt brave enough to ask what had really happened between her mum and dad.

Her mum looked at her. "What really happened? I was just sixteen when I first met your dad. It was up at the rugby club. He seemed to have so much style. 'Cause he was already on the boats, he was earning good money. He seemed the man I dreamed of. I fell in love with him, and he seemed to fancy me…" Gemma looked across the table at her mother. With her hair down tonight – not in a tight bun for the supermarket – her make-up and her earrings glittering in the candlelight, she could almost see the girl her father had fallen for.

Her mother smiled back at her. "The first few years were good. Your dad was working regular and the money – good money – kept coming in. But then the Scottish boats and the Spaniards started fishing nearer and nearer inshore with smaller mesh nets that caught the young fish – so the catches got less and, of course, so did his earnings. And your dad couldn't take it – couldn't take it that he wasn't providing for us, so the rows started." Gemma thought she saw a tear in the corner of her mother's eyes. "And after one particularly bad row –" Gemma wanted to ask if he'd hit her mum, but was afraid to know that he definitely had "– he stormed out and next I heard he was down in Newlyn working on the bigger boats. Well, I just kept trying to keep the house going and bring you up. After a bit, he seemed to be doing OK. He'd come back the odd weekend or couple of days between trips, and I almost got used to that way of life…"

"And then what happened?" Gemma asked.

"Well, the calls got less frequent and the trips home kept being put off, till one day he rang and said he'd be sailing in the next day or two, but could I get down to Newlyn? I said 'Yes' and left you with your Nan." She paused while the waitress – a girl who'd been at school with Gemma – brought the coffee over.

"I took the train to Penzance and the bus down to Newlyn. He seemed really pleased to see me, so we went off to a pub for a meal. He seemed pretty wound up, knocking back the beer, but then your father had always liked a drink. He was telling me how much he'd missed me and how he'd be coming home as soon as possible, when this woman walked in, went up to the bar and kept staring at us. She had a low-cut dress on and she kept on staring, so I knew – and I told him we had to go. He didn't want to, so I stood up – but I couldn't get back to Fishertown because it was so late, so I went back to his place and stayed the night, but I didn't let him near me. He kept saying 'Why not?' but I didn't even bother to answer; I was so angry. And the next morning – it was a Sunday – I walked down to the bus stop in the square and it was raining; there wasn't a soul around, except all those seagulls."

"Oh, mum," was all Gemma could think to say. Her mum smiled at her "But I tell you one thing, young eighteen-year old Gemma – your dad, for all his faults, knew class when he saw it and he'd be proud of you."

Gemma's eyes filled with tears, while at the same time she felt ridiculous, crying at praise from a father who had deserted her.

When she got her head clear, she saw the waitress was bringing two glasses of champagne across. "Roy says with the compliments of the house on your birthday, Gemma." Her mother lifted her glass. "To my beautiful daughter."

When the bill came, Gemma tried to pay for the meal but her mother wouldn't hear of it. "What do you think I work all those hours in the supermarket for?" she said, as she pushed Gemma's money away.

They walked home. Her mother had to work in the morning. Gemma did not feel at all tired, so she decided to go out for a breath of fresh air. She went down to the seafront, where courting couples walked arm in arm.

She thought of her mother on that visit to Newlyn and she wondered if she herself would ever marry. If she did – she'd once been on a school trip to St Germans and she'd always thought she'd like to be married in the old Celtic cathedral there, in the coloured half-light from its medieval stained-glass windows – but would she have any better luck than her Mum? Adam – she remembered his last words before he left about coming back to get her. She wanted to hold him to her, feel his body close up to hers; and she hoped, one more time, that he hadn't found a new girlfriend up in London, someone far more sophisticated and up with the latest fashions than she would ever be – but he had rung to say he should be able to get home for Christmas. Perhaps, if it was fine weather, they'd get *Periwinkle* out of her winter wraps and sail up the West River between the banks of rustling trees – or just walk through the woods together, and get out some daft costumes to celebrate the New Year, and dance on the old bridge at midnight.

Two days later, Gemma got the bus back to the Beacon for the early shift. It was Sunday and she went with Terry and George to St Keverne. Terry now joined in the singing and prayers. Gemma looked at him along the pew. It was strange – he looked younger now than when she first knew him. But George – she worried about him; his chest was definitely worse and his breathing more laboured and panting.

They came out into the white warmth of the autumn sunshine and started to walk through the fields. At one point, before the path started descending to Lantern Beach, the landscape opened and they could see the cliff beneath them and the calm blue sea.

They stopped. Below stretched the same seascape Gemma had seen from her bike just a few months before.

They heard wingbeats and looked up to see a flock of white geese with grey wingtips, flying strongly. They watched as the V-formation got smaller as they sped south over the sea. "Sensible animals," said George. "Following the sun."

Chapter Seventeen

On Lantern Beach

One morning, later that week, a typed notice was circulated to all staff asking them to attend a meeting in the Lookout that afternoon. The bare minimum of staff were left to keep an eye on the residents.

Gemma was uneasy. Typed instructions were so unlike the way the Beacon worked. "What do you think it's about?" she asked Barbara and Rose.

"Looks bad to me," said Rose.

"I'm not so sure," said Barbara. "The last place I worked at, these meetings were just to tell us about important changes in the way the unit was to be run. And what it always seemed to mean was that we were to do what we were already doing but call it by a different name. And if you didn't call it by its new name, the managers used to get terribly cross." Her joking didn't reassure Rose or Gemma. The memory of the evening she had found Mrs O'Halloran crying flickered uneasily through Gemma's mind.

They went up into the Lookout. It was crowded. Gemma hadn't quite realized how many staff it took to run the Beacon.

The room had been arranged so that there was a space between where the staff sat and three chairs facing them on a small raised platform.

At the appointed time, Mrs O'Halloran and two men in suits and ties – strangers – came in, and took their seats.

Mrs Halloran stood up. She began. "Thank you all for coming. We wanted to talk to you before we tell the residents. I have with me two of the directors of the Foundation." She gave their names. "They have spent the last few days in lengthy and intensive discussion with the County Council and have some bad news for us all. I'll hand over to the Financial Director to explain."

The room had gone very quiet and tense.

One of the two strangers stood up. "I want to thank you all for the fantastic work that Beacon House does, for the high quality of care that you all have helped to create. And I think you know that this level of care is far higher than most comparable homes provide. But the downside is that such quality costs more. Up to now, the County Council has been willing to pay this extra cost. But, for the next financial year, it has now decided to cut its contribution back to the legal minimum and we cannot get any guarantees from the Council as to when in the future any variation to this flat rate of payment might be allowed. So each week, each month, we would be running up debts at the Beacon. Now the people who started this Foundation wanted us to put our money into care, not the bank, which means there is not much in the way of reserves. So the cost of keeping Beacon House open would rapidly create unbearable financial strains on the Foundation."

Someone in the audience gave a small cry, "No…".

Someone else called out, "Haven't these people got any rights? Haven't they got the right to a home?"

The director said wearily, "I'm an accountant, not a lawyer. My guess is the Council is hoping we'll keep Beacon House open, and if we can't, they'll find places for our residents anywhere they have vacancies, wherever that might be. But no, they've no legal right to stay here."

There was a silence – the silence of dread. Rose had gone pale. While she had been listening to the announcement, she had squeezed her mouth tightly against her teeth and now a drop of blood was forming on her bottom lip. Barbara had wrapped her arms around herself and was rocking. She was moaning, "No, no, oh no."

Someone shouted, "Moving them will kill them." The three people on the platform looked at each other. The two men seemed paralysed by the anger and pain in the room.

Mrs O'Halloran rose. She spoke quickly. "This means that, as things stand, the Beacon will close in three months."

Some staff did not appear to understand what she had said, but Gemma heard and understood. She had to get out of the meeting. She stood up. Mrs O'Halloran saw her leaving, and softly and helplessly called out, "Gemma." Their eyes caught for an instant, but Gemma could only look at her without acknowledging her. Mrs O'Halloran winced. Gemma ran down the stairs and along the corridor. In her mind's eye, she saw Mrs Bennett as she lay dying; and she heard her words, the night after the party, echo inside her head: "We must protect the good." She ran onto the beach and, almost fainting, stumbled. She put out her hands to save herself but was not quick enough. Her face hit a stone as she fell and then she lay still in the sand.

The residents, hearing the commotion in the room above and outside, came to the south window and pressed their faces against it.

Beatrice and Tom had seen Gemma fall and went to her. Together, with difficulty, they raised her prostrate body, her arms still outstretched, and supported her on their shoulders. Blood trickled down from the cut in her forehead and made a red rivulet in the yellow sand that covered her face.

For a long time they stood holding her, and it was as if she had lost her speech. But gradually they heard a whispered, "They do not know what they are doing." A soft "No," and then the word was spoken again, louder this time like the moaning of a rising wind at night; and turning, wrenching her body toward the blind sea, she screamed with all her might, "No, no, no." Then, pulling Tom and Beatrice to her, and swinging them round towards the other residents, she said more softly but with a fierce determination, "The Beacon will not die."

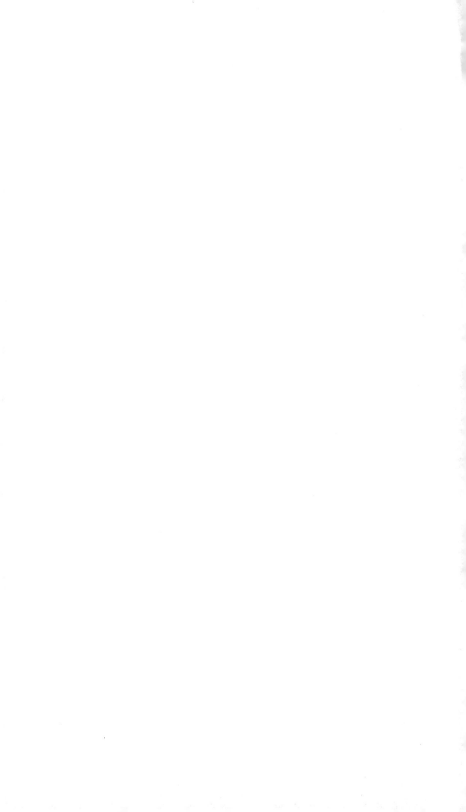